Pregnancy Peace of Mind

NINE STRATEGIES FOR PREGNANT WOMEN, FIRST TIME MOMS AND NEW PARENTS

K. DAVIS-REID

B3K Publishing Inc.

Contents

Introduction

First, congratulations! There are very few moments in any mother's life that compare to when she sees a positive pregnancy test for the first time. With this realization comes a flood of emotions. From the excitement that comes with the news and the wonder and bewilderment when it finally dawns that you are now responsible for the little life growing inside you, to the anticipation and joy of this beautiful season of your life and the excitement of sharing the news with loved ones. These are things you'll never forget.

As soon as the initial joy wears off, your excitement might transition to overdrive quickly – the urge to protect your child at all costs, do everything to make sure they are healthy, and the desire to know and learn everything perfectly right here, right now. This rush of emotions is followed by a flood of questions and long hours of endless google searches.

A recent study done by OnePoll survey reports that expectant and new mothers spend up to eight weeks or approximately 1,400 hours online worrying about and researching baby-related questions during the first year. That's a lot of hours spent worrying, but it sure comes with the territory. It's true what they say; show me a pregnant or new mom, and I'll show you someone who has researched *"how big the baby is at 'x' weeks," "remedies for morning sickness," "can my baby hear me"* or *"should I talk to the baby?"*

The same study showed that pregnant and new mothers did approximately 300 online searches. That's almost one Google search a day. The primary concerns of expectant mothers highlighted by the study were the baby's and mothers' overall health, such as coping with and inducing labor, recovery after delivery, how to have a safe pregnancy, baby's growth, milestones, nutrition and diet, sleep, allergies and how to combat lingering fears.

Obviously, the OnePoll study didn't keep tabs on how often pregnant mothers ask questions on social media platforms, group chats, or the endless phone calls to their mothers and doctor visits. So yes, once you are pregnant, worrying becomes a full-time job. While many of us wish it wasn't this way, the reality is that worry-free pregnancy and parenting don't exist.

Looking back at the two times I was pregnant with my boys; I realize just how overwhelmed I was. I would wake my husband up in the middle of the night to go through hundreds of to-do lists and millions of what-if scenarios. Even worse is that the first pregnancy didn't and couldn't prepare me for the second one. No two pregnancies are alike. I had very different pregnancies and post-pregnancies experiences with both.

My husband and I watched millions of baby and pregnancy-related videos; we researched extensively what happens during each trimester and examined multiple pain management techniques and interventions for live births. We wrote detailed plans, took numerous parenting classes, and prepared ourselves mentally for life during and after pregnancy. I ate, exercised, and napped as I waited for our little miracle. Maybe I was – you know – a little dramatic, I don't know. But, hey, pregnancy is a big deal, and the need for constant reassurance and endless checks are normal.

A recent Canadian study reports significant neurological changes that a mother's brain undergoes during pregnancy, which would explain the persistent worry. Parts of your brain responsible for regulating emotions, empathy, and maternal motivation grow significantly during pregnancy. Even after birth, your desire to take care of the baby remains.

These changes explain the constant Googling.

There is an endless stream of information – and of course, misinformation out there. Think family, friends, the internet, books, and unsolicited advice from strangers and random people. If you aren't careful, you'll suffer from information overload sooner than you think. It's a relief that pregnancy takes nine months, so you have a lot of time to prepare, adjust and plan.

But what if you weaned yourself off of "Dr. Google" a little?

Experts from the University of Waterloo have come out strongly to warn about the dangers of trusting "Dr.

Google" blindly. They argue that google can leave you feeling more confused and less informed than the first time you went in. In another study, medics and researchers reported that close to half of all medical-related google searches could leave you feeling like you just had a cancer diagnosis.

Who wants to add such worries on top of everything already happening?

I have written this book to provide expectant mothers like you with accurate, relevant, and reliable information and guidance. My goal is to help you stay healthy, find support, locate excellent prenatal care, learn about your nutritional options, understand the importance of maternal care and give you advice that reflects your preferences and helps you prioritize your child.

Your body is doing amazing things by the day. It can be a little overwhelming, but it's pretty darn cool. As part of a small, local support group for pregnant women, I hear inspirational stories of first-time moms who start the journey scared and unsure but fall in love with the tiny human they have created once they understand the process. Every week, these women share their experiences, fears, struggles, and concerns about pregnancy. Many are usually excited to meet their children. Like you, they wonder who they will be and what they'll be like: their personalities, dreams, and goals.

I know you want a safe pregnancy so that your baby can develop into a healthy human who can flourish outside your body's protective boundaries once they are born. Having had two vaginal deliveries with and without the assistance of pain relief, I can relate to your concerns. I believe I am well informed to provide valuable insight to you and other fearful and misinformed pregnant mothers.

Many women will tell you scary stories of the countless hours they spent in labor, their pain, and the number of stitches they got. Most of them forget to mention that the most memorable, beautiful moment of your life is about to happen. I come from a big family and have garnered the experience, knowledge & understanding to know that no pregnancy is the same. However, most women agree that whatever it takes to feel the final push and lay eyes on their baby for the first time brings more wonder, excitement, joy, and pride than they've ever felt in their whole life.

Seeing my two boys for the first time was one of the happiest moments of my life. I have asked my husband about it, and he has the same opinion. I love children, and whenever I pass a pregnant mother on the street, I can't help but admire them for a split second. I look at them in awe, knowing that they are about to experience one of the best days of their lives. For these reasons, and many others, I decided to write this book to offer/share insightful information that I wish I had known during both of my pregnancies with you and that pregnant woman down the street.

The truth is, you don't relive the excitement of being a first-time mom twice. You might as well empower yourself with knowledge and take advantage of the experience.

I would say pregnancy is an eye-opening experience. It's at this point where you must examine your finances, diet, relationship, fitness level, and health and make necessary adjustments. Prenatal care becomes critical during pregnancy. It's important to seek necessary medical help or manage existing health issues. In Chapters 1, 4, and 6, I will show you how to ensure you have a healthy pregnancy for yourself and the baby through diet, nutrition, fitness, and exercise.

Pregnancy is a demanding, life-changing process. You may have fears and concerns about childbirth. Chapter

2 highlights all the strategic ways to cope and prepare yourself for the baby. As you go through this journey, you'll find that you desire a support system. You can reach out to other pregnant or new mothers and learn from their experiences. This is an excellent opportunity to build a support system that you can lean on even after your baby is born.

Moving on to childbirth. How will you deal with labor? How do you know you are in labor? Would you rather have a natural birth or c-section? How will your partner help? What pain medicines would you consider? Chapters 7 and 8 describe everything you need to know about labor and childbirth.

Pregnancy and childbirth are beautiful, but the process may not always be perfect. Chapter 9 provides essential information on what you should expect. It highlights what is expected during childbirth, warning signs and when you should call a doctor.

Many emotions and feelings about your relationships and life may resurface as you prepare for motherhood. You may have many questions about your relationship with your parents, their relationship, and its impact on your parenting. Your partner may feel the same. You can take this time to mend fences, work on broken relationships, strengthen existing ones and be clear about your boundaries so you can be a mother on your terms.

Maybe you and your partner are thinking about the huge responsibility ahead. You want to prepare yourself physically, emotionally, and spiritually for the incredible parenting journey. Pregnancy presents an opportunity for you to talk about your expectations and find ways to learn how to be good parents. Think parenting classes, books, or asking friends and relatives about their parenting journey.

Maybe you are an obsessive researcher, or you are clueless. Consider this book your pregnancy and postpartum blueprint. This book will give you a detailed action plan that sets you up for the next nine months and beyond, so you can focus on the more critical pregnancy issues. My goal is to keep you empowered, informed, and knowledgeable in your pregnancy and the first few months after your baby's birth.

Let's turn the page and prepare for the arrival of this baby!

CHAPTER ONE

Guide to a Safe Pregnancy

P regnancy is a life-changing experience that begins as soon as the test comes back positive. Your baby starts to grow, and significant changes in your body, lifestyle, and emotions come with that. As you watch all these things happen, you may have many questions about what to expect. You may be wondering, *"At what point will I get my first ultrasound?", "What should I expect at each stage of fetal development?", "When will I feel the first kick," "what prenatal tests should I expect and at what point?"* among other things.

Every pregnancy is unique, and the details of how it affects the body vary from one individual to the next. Pregnancies can also differ for the same mother, so they have different experiences with different babies. The symptoms also vary, with some going for a few weeks or months compared to other temporary discomforts. However, there are certain stages of pregnancy every mother goes through in their journey.

Stages of pregnancy

Many people assume pregnancy is a nine-month journey. This concept is true to a certain degree because you'll be pregnant for around nine months. Even so, your pregnancy starts from the onset of your last cycle. This is normally two or three weeks before the actual conception date. As you can imagine, most people won't remember the first day of their last menses – and that is fine.

If you were to count your weeks from the first day of your last period, it would mean that you are already four weeks pregnant on the day you were supposed to have your next period. If it's been two weeks since your monthlies were due, you are already six weeks pregnant. Looking at it this way, you would conclude that your pregnancy will be a 40-week journey.

Your doctor will calculate the total length of your pregnancy using the 40-week concept. This estimation is accurate for the most part, but you should always keep in mind that estimation is all that it is. Your baby will arrive when they are ready, and all you have to do is wait patiently.

The 40 weeks are divided into three stages – first, second and third trimester. Each trimester is around 12-13 weeks apart. Every trimester brings new changes as the baby grows and your body tries to keep up.

Many experts have even suggested that the medical community acknowledge "fourth trimesters." The fourth trimester would mean the 12 weeks following birth. This is a crucial moment, too, as your baby tries to adjust to "normal" life outside the womb, and you are just starting to cope with the realities of being a new mom.

What happens during the trimesters?

First trimester - Week 1-13

Many mothers experience wild symptoms during their first trimester. The body slowly adjusts to hormonal changes associated with pregnancy. It's still too early for the pregnancy to show physically during the first few weeks of your first trimester, but believe it or not, many things are happening "behind the scenes."

Week 1-2

Week 1 describes the week of your last menstrual cycle. Week 2 is the week immediately after that. You don't know it yet, but your body is making necessary changes for two main events – ovulation and fertilization.

It's incredible to think that the countdown to your baby's birth starts with ovulation, way before fertilization occurs. Think of these two weeks as the last moments before you have a new tenant in the "house." You aren't exactly pregnant, but you might as well start acting like you are. Quit smoking and alcohol, and start working towards a healthier diet.

Once the egg is released, it will travel down the fallopian tube, where fertilization occurs. Fertilization takes place near the end of the second week.

Symptoms to look out for during weeks 1-2

- Increased production of cervical mucus
- Temperature spikes and dips before and during ovulation

Week 3-4

Congratulations. You are officially pregnant, but it will be a while until you can confirm this with a pregnancy test. The fertilized egg forms a cluster of cells and grows rapidly. The egg splits into two cells 30 hours after fertilization. The two cells divide into 16 cells by the third day following conception. As the cells divide, they travel through the fallopian tube and arrive in the uterus four days after fertilization. After fertilization, the egg divides

5

into thousands of cells, some of which will form the embryo and others placenta. However, the cells are no bigger than the full stop at the end of this sentence. Tiny, but don't underestimate their power. Exactly seven days after fertilization, these microscopic cells will burrow into the lining of your uterus, a process known as implantation. Now, you have a "cake baking in the oven."

So, is it a boy or a girl? It's too soon for modern medical equipment to tell, but your baby's sex has been determined already. If the winning sperm carries an X chromosome, you'll have a girl, and if it carries a Y chromosome, you'll have yourself a cute little boy. After conception, your body will experience a huge surge in hormone production which may manifest in an increased sense of smell – one of the first signs of pregnancy.

Chorionic gonadotropin hormone (hCG) is one of the first hormones the body releases following conception. This hormone is what the home pregnancy tests detect because it appears in your urine around a week after you miss your period.

Increased estrogen levels, hCG, and other hormones will manifest as vomiting and waves of nausea, famous or infamously known as morning sickness. Morning sickness usually occurs early on in your pregnancy. The name "morning sickness" might be a little misleading,

though. These symptoms may occur at any hour of the day, morning, midday, evening, etc.

At week four, the baby is no larger than the tiniest grain of rice you've ever seen. The cells divide rapidly and start the complex exercise of creating critical body systems such as the digestive system, nervous system, internal organs, skin, hair, cells, and eyes. The amniotic and yolk sac form around these cells. The yolk sac is later absorbed into the baby's digestive system.

Symptoms to look out for in weeks 3-4

- You may feel some pressure in the lower abdominal region. It's normal to feel mild cramping without bleeding.

- Weird metallic taste. This is also normal because of the hormones wreaking havoc in your system.

- Tender breasts

Week 5-6

At this point, you've officially stepped into your second week of pregnancy. You can take a pregnancy test at five weeks because hCG levels are high enough to give a positive result. You may also feel a little tired and nauseous. There is so much growing to do to become a baby, right? The heart, lungs, stomach, and other systems have to grow from nothing. At five weeks, your little human's heart and the circulatory system slowly develop. The neural tube that eventually becomes your baby's nervous system slowly grows.

Since the circulatory system and its accompanying organs develop first, you may hear a faint heartbeat on an ultrasound at week five. The baby is around 3-5mm long, still very tiny; they may be as big as an orange seed now. Right now, these faint heartbeats come from two small heart tubes that will eventually fuse to form a normal heart. The spinal cord and brain, which form the neural tubes, haven't sealed, but that quickly happens in the sixth week.

In week six, the embryo starts to look more like a baby. Little cheeks, jaws, and a little head start to form. Now you are feeling completely pregnant. The baby has been releasing hormones to stop menstruation, so you've missed your period, your bathroom visits have doubled, and you experience heartburn and nausea time and again.

At six weeks, the baby has grown to the size of a sweet pea. The ear canals are developing. At this time, the heart takes on a full 110 beats per minute, and the liver, lungs and kidneys are developing too.

Symptoms to look out for in weeks 5-6

- Frequent urination

- Heartburn

- Indigestion

- Production of excess saliva

- Nausea

- Fatigue

Week 7-8

Let's take a moment to enjoy a fun fact: did you know that at this point, the fetus is 10,000 times bigger than when you started this journey? They are about ¼- ½ inches long; more like the size of a blueberry. Still small, right?

That may be the case, but your little one's heart is growing bigger by the day. They are growing 100 brain cells per minute because the head is the main focus of growth at seven weeks. Isn't that great news for a blossoming genius? Limbs start to form, but at this early stage, they look like tiny webbed buds. These limbs will lengthen soon and divide into shoulders, limbs, hands, knees and feet.

Other external features such as mouth, tongue, eyes, ears, and thin eyelids are forming. Tiny kidneys have developed too, ready to start their important job of removing wastes. The kidneys are especially important right now because the placenta has already burrowed into the uterine wall and will soon start to transport oxygen and nutrients from your bloodstream to the baby. These nutrients must also be removed from the baby's system as waste.

At week eight, the baby has grown from a little blueberry to the size of a raspberry. Following the 8th week period, the baby grows at a rate of one millimeter every day, making it quite the challenge to estimate the actual size. The growth isn't limited to height. They are coming from every direction – arms, legs, and an actively growing spinal cord which may look like a tail at first glance.

Tiny toes and fingers start to grow from the "webbed limbs" and the tiny embryo starts to look more like a baby. Even better, your baby's limbs start to twitch and make spontaneous movements, even though you are still less likely to notice. Soon enough, the limbs will be strong enough for that incredible first kick. The heartbeat has increased to an incredible 150-170 beats per minute.

There will be a significant increase in amniotic fluid and womb size to accommodate the growing baby.

Symptoms to look out for in weeks 7-8

- Recurrent morning sickness following the expansion of the uterus. (Fortunately, morning sickness reduces significantly around the 12th-14th week, so you'll get some relief soon.)

- Aversions

- Constipation may occur

- Bloating

- Fatigue

- Gas

- Vomiting

- Nausea

- Vaginal discharge

Week 9-10

Think of a medium-sized green olive; yes, that's how big your baby is at week nine. The facial features including mouth, tongue and eyes are still growing. The embryo can also move about at this point, thanks to some tiny muscles already in place. The arms and legs are making slow movements, but you won't feel them yet. What's more, the liver is actively producing blood cells.

Other critical body organs including the brain, heart, lungs, and kidneys continue to grow. While it's still too early to feel things, it's not too early to hear them. The heart is large and strong enough to be heard through an ultrasound. Don't freak out if you can't hear the baby's heartbeat through the ultrasound yet. Maybe the doppler can't find its target because they are turned back or hiding in a "distant" corner of your uterus.

At week ten, the baby finally graduates from an embryo to a fetus. The baby grows rapidly at this point. Now, they could be around 2.5cm long, think of something the size of a prune. Most body organs are fully formed. Even the "webbed limbs" are now fully evolved toes and fingers.

The arms have little elbows which can be flexed, while the ankles and knees have already been formed on the legs.

Didn't think you'd get a visit from the tooth fairy? Well, your baby's first teeth are slowly forming below their gums, but you'll never see them until they are around six months old. The kidney is actively removing wastes in the form of urine, and digestive juices are being produced by the stomach. If it's a boy, they are producing testosterone too.

Symptoms to look out for in weeks 9-10

- Cravings and aversions

- Fatigue

- Vomiting

- Nausea

- Indigestion

- Bloating

- Gas

- Heartburn

- Headaches

- Dizziness

- Fainting

- Visible veins on your breasts and stomach. They will disappear soon

- Pains around the belly. This is normal because the ligaments are being pulled from either side of your stomach as the baby grows.

Weeks 11-12

Your baby is busy growing in the 11th week. Now they weigh around ¼ of an ounce; think something like a large strawberry. Tiny hair follicles are starting to sprout on your baby's crown and the whole body. Remember the webbed-like feet and toes? You can say goodbye to them because they have been replaced by individual toes and fingers. Obviously, these tiny toes and fingers will need nails, which will slowly develop in the next few weeks. You better add a nail clipper to your shopping list now.

It's still impossible to tell the baby's gender, but the ovaries are developing if it is biologically female. At 11 weeks your baby starts to develop unique human characteristics like the rest of us. Their nipples are visible, the mouth has a tongue and palate, the feet and hands face forward distinctly, and their tiny nose has open passages.

The baby can stretch, move, roll and change positions frequently.

At 12 weeks, the tiny human inside your womb weighs a full ounce; in size, think limes. It might not show and you might not believe it, but the baby's size has more than doubled in the last three weeks. The 12-week mark is an important milestone. At this stage, the development of body organs is almost coming to an end. Many systems are fully formed by this point, but there's still a lot of maturing to be done.

The next phase is critical because your baby's systems are set to mature over the next 28 weeks. Most important is the digestive system, whose contractions start to mature in preparation of food outside the womb.

Symptoms to look out for in weeks 11-12

- Excessive production of saliva

- Headaches

- Bloating

- A heightened sense of smell

- More bathroom trips

- Fatigue

- Gas

Week 13

You've made it to the last week of your first trimester. The fetus is around 7cm in length; think something like a lemon. External sex organs are fully formed and an ultrasound can reveal the baby's sex at this stage. The fetus can move around the womb vigorously during the 13th

week. The hair follicles have hair growing in them while the arms and feet grow their own little bones as well.

As the baby grows, their nutritional needs must keep up too. For this reason, the placenta continues to grow the baby's needs. The intestines also move to your baby's abdomen, their natural and permanent location. Up to this point, the intestines were growing in the umbilical cord's cavity. If the fetus is biologically female, they'll grow little prostate glands. If they are biologically female, their ovaries will slowly shift to the pelvic area from the abdomen.

Even more interesting is, the baby's vocal cords also develop in the 13th week. Now they'll have a little voice to cry, laugh and sing when the time is right.

Symptoms to look out for in week 13

- Cravings and aversions

- Heartburn

- Increased energy levels

- Dizziness

- Faintness

- Veins become visible

- Indigestion

- Constipation

Second trimester

Week 14-15

The baby grows rapidly in the second trimester. This week, they weigh around 2 ounces and measure around 3-4 inches long; think a navel orange or the size of your clenched fist. The baby moves constantly but you won't feel the movements yet. It will be a few months of waiting till your baby stands on two feet once they are born, but believe me they are doing it right now, without any help at all.

Since the neck has grown a little longer than the last time you checked, the baby can now hold their head up in an erect position. Their little eyebrows are filled with hair and their eyes are fully developed, though still tightly shut my eyelids. The baby has vocal cords, and you'd be surprised to learn that they can cry, albeit mutely. The roof over your baby's mouth develops too and they have minimal digestive system activity too.

You may start to look pregnant at this point, and that's okay, because the baby is growing rapidly by the time you hit the 15-week mark. They are as big as a pear now, can weigh around 4 inches and are approximately 4.5 inches in length. At 15 weeks, the ears are perfectly placed on each side of their head and the eyes have finally moved to the front of their face.

Meanwhile, the baby starts to develop critical survival skills such as breathing and sucking. They can move their legs and arms, curl their toes, and kick, but since it weighs nothing more than just a few pounds, you won't feel it just yet.

Symptoms to look out for in weeks 14-15

- Heartburn

- Dizziness

- Indigestion

- Headaches

- Belly pain

- Varicose veins

- Forgetfulness

- Breast tenderness

- You feel a little energetic

- Blocked nasal cavity

- Vomiting

- Nausea

Week 16-17

At 16 weeks, the baby weighs around 4 ounces and is approximately 5 inches long. The baby can comfortably stretch her back and straighten out its head because their backbone and tiny back muscles have more strength. Not only can the baby move its eyes from left to right, but they can also make a few facial expressions including frowns, squints, etc.

The baby's eyelids are sealed shut, but they can perceive light, which would explain the eye movements. Eyebrows and eyelashes are fully developed and the little tongue has taste buds.

Now, here's the more interesting bit:

The fetus's ears are fully developed and the tiny bones inside them are in place. While the baby is more likely to hear distinct sounds at around 18 weeks, they can perceive the sound of your voice faintly.

Fun fact
Did you know that a baby can recognize a tune that was sung to them while they were still in the womb even after they are born? Keep this in mind every time you sing them a song.

17 weeks into the pregnancy, the baby will weigh around 5 ounces, approximately the size of your palm. Your baby perfects most of its survival reflexes at 17 weeks. These include breathing, swallowing and sucking. Most importantly however, your baby is on the road toward

developing distinctive individual characteristics. In the next few weeks, their fingers and toes will develop unique patterns, also known as fingerprints and toe prints.

Symptoms to look out for in weeks 16-17

- Stretchmarks

- Lots of back pain

- Headaches

- Increased appetite

- Heartburn

- Increases breast tissue

- Constipation

- You may suffer from bleeding gums

- Vaginal discharge

Week 18-19

The baby weighs approximately 5-6 ½ ounces in week 18. They will be big enough for you to feel them roll, turn, kick and punch in the next few weeks. Along with that, the baby's nervous system is flourishing and forming complex connections. The nerves in the brain are maturing, and with them, complex senses such as touch, smell, sight, etc.

At 18 weeks, your baby's hearing is fully developed, and they can hear you distinctly from this point on.

At week 19, the baby will weigh a little over half a pound. Your baby's skin is also covered by vernix caseosa and lanugo. Lanugo is fine hair, while vernix caseosa is a cheesy varnish, both of which are meant to protect your baby while they are still in the womb.

Symptoms to look out for in weeks 18-19

- Bloating

- Fetal movement

- Swelling in your ankles and feet

- Cramping, especially around the legs

- Bleeding gums

- Backaches

- Blocked nasal cavity

- Constipation

- Increase in appetite

Weeks 20-21

Your baby is stacking up the weights by week 20 and is well over 10 ounces and around 6½ inches in height. They can hear muffled sounds because their ears are fully functional. Their fingers have prints too. They might be bigger, but there is still so much room in the womb, so they can easily twist and turn when they want to.

By this time, an ultrasound can show your baby's gender even though their external genitals are far from fully developed. If the baby is biologically female, the uterus will have formed entirely by this stage. The vaginal canal is also in its initial stages of development. Their immature ovaries have millions of primitive eggs.

If the baby is biologically male, they'll have to wait a few more weeks for the scrotum to form before the testicles can permanently take their position.

At 21 weeks, the baby weighs 11-12 ½ ounces; think something like a giant banana now. You'll feel their occasional twisting, turning, and kicking. What's even more surprising is that whatever you eat from week 21, your baby might "eat" it too. Your baby swallows tiny bits of amniotic fluid every day for hydration, nutrition, and "swallowing classes."

The baby's taste buds are fully functional, and every day, they get to taste what's on the menu. It's worth noting that what your baby tastes in the amniotic fluid differs depending on what you ate on that specific day.

Here's an exciting fact; introducing your baby to certain foods while still in the womb makes them eager to taste the same food after birth? If you want them to learn healthy habits, you may as well start introducing them to healthy foods right now.

Symptoms to look out for in weeks 20-21

- Swelling in the feet and ankles

- Headaches

- Cramping around the legs

- Heartburn

- Indigestion

- Your navels may protrude

- Baby movements

- Fast-growing nails

Weeks 22-23

Your baby weighs a little over a pound and approximately 11inches at 21 weeks; think a tiny doll. Your baby can taste well at this point, hear, perceive light, and move their eyes from side to side.

This week, their sense of touch will be polished too. On top of that, they'll have fully developed muscles, fingers, and hands to grab things, and they have a firm grip. Too bad there is still nothing to hold in the womb.

About their perception of light, the womb is dark, but if you were to shine a flashlight on your belly, which you can also try, they'd be able to perceive it. The baby can also hear everything that's going on in your system; your heartbeat, stomach sounds, your circulating blood, and voice.

Your baby will start to add significant weight at 23 weeks. By the time you get to the 27th week, they might have doubled their weight. Hopefully, your doctor can find their heartbeat, not just with a doppler but with a stethoscope. The heartbeat might be a little hard to find, so don't worry if it doesn't happen just yet.

Symptoms to look out for in weeks 22-23

- Indigestion

- Stretch marks as the baby continues to grow

- Cramping, especially around your legs

- Constipation

- Your navel continues to protrude

Weeks 24-25

The one-pound mark hasn't been surpassed yet, but your baby gains around 6 ounces every week, slowly but surely. All body organs grow, and fats are deposited under the baby's skin. The baby's facial features are fully formed, and they've also grown hair, lashes, and brows. You'd be intrigued to learn that the hairs have no pigment, so it's impossible to tell what color of hair they'll have.

Even more fascinating is that the baby can hear your voice and your partner's voice, sounds such as loud music, the honking of a car, and everything else happening inside your body.

At 25 weeks, the baby has added an extra ½ a pound and would weigh 1½ pounds now. The baby can start practicing breathing movements now that the nose and nostrils have started working. While there is no air in the womb for the baby to breathe, the practice is what counts.

Symptoms to look out for in weeks 24-25

- You may feel some tingling in your hands

- Your hair grows super-fast

- Your legs start to feel restless

- You may snore

- Heartburn

- Indigestion

Week 26-27

By the time you hit the 26th-week mark, your baby will have added enough weight to weigh around 2 pounds. There is still enough room for them to grow in the womb, but they may start to feel a little confined at this stage. Now, they have less room to move around.

Your baby can't see much from the uterus, but by the 26th week, the retinas in their eyes are almost mature enough for them to focus on objects once they are born. The uterus is dark, but since they can perceive light, try shining a flashlight through your stomach to see if you'll get some movements. Even better, your baby's levels of brain waves are so strong that they can respond to specific triggers by moving, kicking, or rolling.

Twenty-seven weeks is an excellent time to start singing or even reading books to your baby. Find some cute lullabies or rhymes that you can put on repeat. The nerves in the baby's ears are mature, and their auditory system is functional. They can hear you sing or read, even though the sounds are still muffled. The taste buds are fully developed, and they can distinguish spicy food from plain food by tasting different flavors in the amniotic fluid.

Do you want to try something exciting? Ask your partner to press their ear on your belly and see if they can hear the baby's heartbeat.

Symptoms to look out for in weeks 26-27

- Blocked nasal cavity

- Your legs feel restless

- Belly itches

- Pains around the belly as the ligaments stretch

- You may experience bleeding gums

- Dizziness

- You may feel faint

- Forgetfulness

- Blurry vision

- Bloating

- You may be a little clumsy

- Migraines

Third trimester

You made it to the third trimester. It's only a few weeks until your bundle of joy arrives. Meanwhile, they must continue growing.

Week 28-29

By week 28, your baby weighs a little over 2 pounds. The body has grown in the last few weeks, and the baby's head looks more proportional to the body now. They are slowly getting into the proper position, headfirst next to the closest exit.

The baby also works on perfecting their survival skills, including breathing, sucking, and coughing, among other things. At 28 weeks, brain wave measurements reveal sleep cycles that may result in dreams.

By the 29th week, the baby weighs between 2-3 pounds and approximately 16 inches in length; think something like a cauliflower. There is still so much weight it needs to add in the next few weeks, but they are very close to their birth weight.

Your baby is in a confined space because they've grown and filled it up, so you'll feel kicks and pokes frequently. Maybe they are stretching? The baby is strong now, which means the movements will be more vigorous and energetic.

Symptoms to look out for in weeks 28-29

- Forgetfulness

- Constipation which may cause hemorrhoids

- Fast-growing nails

- Heartburn

- Blocked nasal cavity

- Melasma

- Indigestion and gas

- Bloating

Week 30-31

From week 30 on, your baby will add approximately half a pound every other week, but now, she weighs around 3 pounds. The baby's brain must also keep up with its body, so it continues to grow faster and pack on its characteristic fold and dips. The folds allow for additional brain tissue, so you have an intelligent baby when they are born.

With the brain in place and fat cells deposited under the baby's skin, the body hair they had in the last few weeks, also known as lanugo, starts to fall off. Another critical development is that your baby's bone marrow is fully functional. It has completely replaced the spleen and different tissues in producing blood cells.

It's been a long journey, but by week 31, your baby weighs well over 3 pounds. The baby's five senses are fully developed, and they are smart enough to process everything going on around them and track light and any signals in the outside world.

Symptoms to look out for in weeks 30-31

- Frequent bathroom visits

- Forgetfulness

- Backaches

- Headaches and migraines

- Clumsiness

- You may have trouble sleeping

- Fatigue

- Constipation

- Bloating

- Swelling around the feet and ankles

- Stretchmarks on your body

Weeks 32-33

The baby has, at this point, most likely taken the "head down" position, getting ready for the big day. The baby weighs approximately 3½ - 4 pounds and spends most of its time sleeping. Don't worry if the baby hasn't flipped to the head-down position; you still have a few weeks left for them to get into the proper position. Besides, many studies have shown that less than 5% of babies assume the bottom down position before birth, which shows how rarely it happens.

The baby will have added another pound in a week so that they weigh at least 4½ pounds by week 33. The baby's movements may feel a little intense and vigorous right now. At this stage, the baby sleeps with its eyes closed and opens them while awake, just like a normal baby would do.

Your uterine walls have stretched out so much that they are thin enough for more light to penetrate, so your baby can quickly tell the difference between night and day. Their pupils can either dilate or constrict depending on their exposure to light. Most importantly, however, your baby's immune system is in place, but they still rely on you to pass them some antibodies until they can develop their own ultimately.

Symptoms to look out for in weeks 32-33

- Your breasts may start to leak with colostrum in preparation for the baby

- Constipation which may cause hemorrhoids

- Cramping around your legs

- You may feel faint or dizzy

- Strong baby movements

- Forgetfulness

- Minor contractions in mothers who've been pregnant before

- Your nails begin to change

- You may experience pains as your ligaments continue to stretch

- You may become a little clumsy

Week 34-35

Your baby probably weighs 5¼ pounds by week 34. Imagine holding a pineapple if you can't get a mental picture of this. That's how big the baby is. If the baby is biologically male, their testicles should be shifting from the abdomen to their permanent position in the scrotum.

The baby's fingertips probably have nails by now, so you better prepare that nail clipper you bought a few weeks ago.

By week 35, the baby's skin is no longer wrinkled because they have fat deposits under them. They are a bit plumper than they were a few weeks ago.

Symptoms to look out for in weeks 34-35

- Swollen feet and ankles

- Headaches

- Constipation

- Cramping around the legs

- Headaches

- Your breasts leak in preparation for the baby

- Sleeping difficulties

- Your hair grows at an alarming rate

- Vaginal discharge

- Rashes

- Light contractions if you are not a first-time mom

- Your veins may become visible

Week 36-37

You now have an approximately 6-pound baby at 36 weeks. However, their growth rate must slow down in the next few weeks, so they aren't too big to pass through the birth canal. You also need to stack up some energy for the heavy task ahead, so their growth may have to wait a little bit right now.

Most systems are mature and fully functional, but a few things may have to wait longer to fully mature. One of them is the baby's digestive system, which might be fully developed, but has never been used because the baby relied on you entirely for their nutritional needs.

Furthermore, the baby's bones and cartilage are still fragile to allow for an easy birth.

On average, the baby would weigh about 6 pounds by week 38. The space in the uterus might be too tight for them to kick, but you may feel them roll, wiggle, and stretch. The fetus has baby mannerisms, including suckling, inhaling, exhaling, blinking, and moving.

Symptoms to look out for in weeks 36-37

- Baby movements

- Frequent bathroom visits

- Constipation which may cause hemorrhoids

- That motherly instinct starts to kick in, and you may begin to nest

- Sleep problems

- Your vaginal discharge may have tiny blood spots

- Pain in the pelvic area

- Forgetfulness

Week 38-39

By week 38, the baby weighs around 7 pounds and is approximately 20 inches in size.

A few changes are being made at week 38, including fine-tuning the nervous system and brain and adding fat deposits under the skin.

At week 39, your baby may weigh approximately 7-pounds and can be referred to as a full-term baby. Minimal changes will occur in your baby's development from this point on.

Symptoms to look out for in weeks 38-39

- Nesting

- Sleeping problems

- Swollen feet and ankles

- Frequent visits to the bathroom

- Diarrhea

- Vaginal mucus

- Minor contractions for non-first-time moms

- Breasts may leak colostrum

- Heartburn

- You may experience pelvic pain from time to time

Week 40

Week 40 marks the official end of your pregnancy journey. The baby weighs around 6-9 pounds at this point. Don't be alarmed if the baby is smaller or bigger than this. Always keep in mind that these numbers are nothing more than approximates. Your baby may be perfectly healthy, even if they are smaller or bigger.

The baby has turned into the head-down position at week 40. The lungs and other systems are fully developed, ready for birth and survival outside the womb.

When they finally arrive, most mothers check the baby's gender to ensure they are either boys or girls like they were told. Once that part is over, you'll realize the baby is still covered with body fluids, including blood and amniotic fluid. Your baby's vision is still in its developmental stages, so you may appear blurry to them, but they will recognize your voice almost instantly. They've been hearing your voice for weeks, remember?

The baby might still be curled in the same fetal position as in the womb. This position is normal. First, that's the position they are familiar with, and secondly, it may take them some time to understand that they are outside the womb and have more room to stretch. That position is also comforting, as it reminds them of the womb.

Symptoms to look out for in week 40

- Sleep difficulties

- Cramps around your legs

- Nesting

- You may experience pelvic pains

- Dilation of the cervix

Weeks 41-42

Studies show that less than 5% of babies arrive on their appointed due date. The same studies show that 10% of babies are born past the expected 40-week mark. You should also remember that maybe the dates were miscalculated, and your baby isn't overdue.

Late arrivals are standard, but you'll get extra attention from the doctor at 42 weeks, just so they are sure everything is fine with the baby. Don't worry if the baby is born with dry, cracked, or wrinkled skin. Remember, the protective layers were shed a while back in preparation for birth. It's okay if they have longer nails and hair or seem more alert.

Symptoms to look out for in week 41

- Frequent bathroom visits

- Pain in the pelvic area

- Dilation of the cervix

- Spotting may occur

- Your breasts may leak with colostrum

- You may have swollen feet and ankles

- Cervical dilation

- Diarrhea

Prenatal appointments

Prenatal care is critical during pregnancy. It's the only way your healthcare provider ensures you are okay and have a healthy pregnancy. You should start your prenatal care as soon as you realize you are pregnant. Make sure you show up for all your appointments even if you are not feeling sick. Starting your prenatal care soon enough is the only way you are guaranteed a healthy baby and pregnancy.

Don't be scared to open up to your caregiver about personal issues. The more the doctor knows, the more likely they are to help you if you have a problem and give you the best care possible. Remember everything you tell them is confidential, so they would never share them with anyone without your permission.

So, how often should you visit a specialist for prenatal care? Here's a schedule that you can follow:

From your 4th week to the 28th week of pregnancy – visit your health care provider at least once a month and get a checkup.

From the 28th week to the 36th week of your pregnancy – visit your healthcare provider at least twice every month and get a checkup.

From your 36th week to the 41st or 42nd week – visit the healthcare provider once a week and get a checkup.

You may be required to show up more if you have any pregnancy-related complications. You can always invite a friend, partner, or family member to your appointments, so you are not alone.

Where to go for prenatal care services

- **Obstetrician/gynecologist**

They are also known as OB/GYNs. They are specialists, well-trained, and experienced in delivering babies and caring for expectant mothers. Find one in your local area and set up your first appointment.

- **Family Nurse Practitioners/Women Health Nurse Practitioners**

They are also FPNs or WHNPs. FNPs are nurses who specialize in taking care of all your family members, while WHNPs are trained to care for women in general, including expectant mothers.

Find one in your local area through their website and set up your first appointment.

- **Certified nurse-midwives**

They are also known as CNMs. CNMs are well-trained in caring for women of all ages, including pregnant women. You can find a certified nurse to work with from the American College of Nurse-Midwives.

- **Maternal-Fetal Medicine specialists**

They are also known as MFMs. MFMs are OBs, but they receive specialized training in nursing women with high-risk pregnancies. Your health care provider may recommend an MFM if they suspect that you may have problems during pregnancy. You can also find an MFM in your local area by visiting the Society for Maternal-Fetal Medicine website.

- **Family doctors**

They are also known as family physicians. They are well-trained and experienced in taking care of all your family needs. They can also take care of your pregnancy needs up to your delivery date.

Emotions & fear

You'll experience sprawling emotions during your pregnancy, and that's okay. Morning sickness aside, you'll have to deal with constant mood swings; you might become fearful or irritable often. This emotional rollercoaster could result from the continuous spikes and dips in hormones, worries about what lies ahead, fear of the unknown, and general physical discomforts resulting from pregnancy.

You may feel low and sad one minute and full of excitement and joy the next. You are not alone in this; it happens to everybody.

Fear and stress associated with pregnancy usually result from uncertainty about the future. You may be asking yourself millions of questions and have very few answers. This may cause anxiety and fear. Many women admit to asking themselves questions such as:

- Is the baby okay at this stage?

- Will I be okay while giving birth?

- Am I ready for motherhood, and will I be good at it?

- How will we manage financially?

- How will the arrival of this baby affect the relationship I have with my partner?

- Will things change?

- Can I have a career after giving birth?

- Will I lose myself in the process of being a mother, or can I still have my own life?

- Will the same problems I had in my last pregnancy happen this time?

- Have I consumed anything that will potentially harm my unborn child?

Body changes will also affect your moods.

Pregnancy changes your body in significant ways, and with that, your emotions too. Some women love the physical changes brought about by pregnancy, while others don't like how they feel or look when they are pregnant. For instance, you may be worried about how much weight you've gained in the last few weeks and how hard you'll have to work to shed it off.

You may also grow tired of the constant feeling of being sick, tired, constipated, nauseous, bloated, etc. Being too tough on yourself while you are pregnant won't help. Maybe you see many pictures of pregnant women living their happy, best lives on social media and in pregnancy magazines, but we all know this is far from reality. Some women don't like how pregnancy affects them, and that's okay.

It's normal to feel unsure, anxious, and unprepared about how everything will turn out. If the negative feelings and sadness don't go away, you can visit or call your healthcare provider and talk to them about the situation. It's good to speak up if you have any problems or worries about your pregnancy.

It's also important to understand that your sex drive might change during pregnancy. How pregnancy and emotions affect your sex life is an experience that is unique to every woman. Some love it; others loath sex when they are pregnant. This is an important subject to discuss with your partner so you are on the same page.

Your sex life may change for so many reasons, for example:

- You may be a little conscious about your body with all the changes happening right now

- You and your partner may be worried about potentially harming the baby while having sex

- You are constantly tired, sick, and too exhausted to have sex

- You and your partner may be anxious about the challenging parenting task ahead

- You might be uncomfortable during sex, so you'd rather not have it

Sex with your partner is safe; it would never hurt your baby. Unless your health care provider has warned you against it, you should refrain from it; the baby will be okay. Speak up about important things; everything you feel, sex, finances, etc.

If your feelings about sex have changed, let your partner know why and if they can help. Don't shut them out. Speaking can diffuse the tension built up over time and reassure your partner. You may even figure out other ways to be intimate without necessarily having sex involved.

How to cope with wild emotions during pregnancy

It's normal to be worried, stressed, anxious, and fearful. There are times you will be happy and excited, but this may not always be the case. Even ordinary people don't feel happy and excited 24/7. Just because you don't feel excited all the time doesn't mean your pregnancy is a mistake or that you don't love your unborn child unconditionally.

Don't feel guilty about what you feel. Don't feel bad that you don't feel happy all the time when everyone is excited about the pregnancy and expects you to feel the same. You feel what you feel, and many mothers will admit that they've felt the same at some point.

So, what can you do to cope with your emotions?

- Speak to someone, a friend, family, or caregiver

- Stay positive, and don't let negativity rob you of your joy. Try your best to stay on top of your game.

- Deal with your stresses one after another

- You may be anxious because you don't have the correct information. Do your research if you must and find accurate opinions and facts.

- Ask for help when you need it.

CHAPTER TWO

Combating your Lingering Fears and Taking Action

Pregnancy can have beautiful and wild moments, whether planned or unplanned. Every mother's experience is unique, which means they'll approach these experiences differently. This also means that there is no one-size-fits-all advice for every pregnant mother. While many pregnancy symptoms cut across, there is a good chance your experiences will differ from your mothers, friends, or sisters.

Asking for and getting advice from friends and family is a "side-effect" of getting pregnant, but keep in mind that whatever works or applies to someone else may not apply or even work for you. This is okay.

Pregnancy and childbirth will be some of the biggest, life-changing moments in your life. There is more to them than shopping for baby clothes and picking a cute little crib. Everything matters; the tiniest details matter, from where you'd like to give birth to who you allow in the room and everything you have in your little hospital bag. For this reason, and many others, you'll have to be physically and mentally prepared for your child's arrival.

Your healthcare provider, midwife, family, and friends will all support you as much as they can during the pregnancy. Still, it's your responsibility to take control of your situation, mentally and physically, so you are well-prepared for your baby's arrival.

Being mentally and physically prepared for childbirth

Mentally

Create a support system

The old phrase, "it takes a village," has never been more relevant than right now. Multiple studies report that a reliable support system during pregnancy directly and positively affects a mother's postpartum health. And that's not even the extent of it. A strong support system reduces the possibility of premature birth, which means you should find your "village" soon, before childbirth.

It's time to think about who's in your corner; it can be your partner, friends, family, women from your newborn care class, psychologists, or trustworthy healthcare providers. Think about everything you need help with and find a willing party to delegate the task to. This way, you'll have more time to rest and prepare for this significant change in your life.

While joining group chats and online pregnancy chat groups on social media might sound like an excellent idea, they might quickly turn into abysses of misinformation, anxiety, and unwelcome judgment. My advice – they can be awesome, but you must be careful.

Understand that reality might be different from expectation

You've seen beautiful pregnant women on social media and magazine covers. These women seem like they are living their best lives. Everyone expects you to have that "pregnancy glow" and unswerving feelings of happiness, gratitude, and joy. The reality might be very different.

Pregnancy might be a wild ride of nausea, vomiting, morning sickness, chronic fatigue, mood swings, restlessness, swollen legs and ankles, diarrhea, and other pregnancy-related symptoms for some women. I hope this isn't your pregnancy story, but don't set the bar too high. Your spirits will not be crushed if things don't turn out as expected. Most women don't get that pregnancy glow widely popularized on social media, and that's okay.

Change is coming, so be prepared for it.

Pregnancy is just the start of many life-altering transitions; it will change your body and life in many positive ways. You'll have to make enormous adjustments for your growing family, emotionally, physically, and financially. You will grow in so many ways and learn amazing things you didn't know about yourself. Exciting as it may sound, many people fear change and are unwilling to embrace it.

Please focus on the positivity of growing a human inside you and the joy of waiting for their arrival. Forget what you think you are missing out on and prepare yourself for the fantastic journey ahead. You might not have time to be the party animal you used to be or hang out with your girls as much as you used to, but this is an opportunity to focus on your relationship with yourself, your partner, and the tiny human growing inside of you.

Speak up

It's normal to feel anxious, worried, and fearful during pregnancy and childbirth. Fortunately, you don't have to and shouldn't bottle in everything you feel. You'll wear yourself and your baby with things that you can solve easily if you do. Speak to your partner, your friend, family, and healthcare professionals. Be open about what you feel; fear, anxiety, joy, worry, and everything relating to pregnancy and childbirth.

This will strengthen the bond with the people you have around you. It is also an excellent way to ensure everyone is on the same page as the big day draws near. Always remember that while the baby is growing inside you for nine months and you know everything you feel, everyone else is simply waiting for you to hand them the bundle of joy once it's born.

Everyone wants to support you and be ready for the baby's arrival, so you must let them in.

Be patient and gentle with yourself.

There are many expectations of women to "bounce back" after childbirth. Many experts have suggested recently that Eastern cultures have always understood the "fourth-trimester" idea. However, women in western countries may not enjoy the luxury of a 12-week postpartum period. Even if they have time and space to do it, some feel like they need to bounce back faster. You'll find them set on working out and starting diets to get their body back.

It's hard to see that your body has changed so much, but you must try and prepare yourself mentally for these changes. Your body will change significantly; after all, a whole human is growing inside you. This isn't something to be ashamed of. It is something to be grateful for.

It's okay to take a break and focus on yourself, the baby, and your mental health. Everyone gives you support, but you should give yourself as much time and support as you need to during pregnancy and after birth.

Physically

Training an exercise

If you were an athlete, you'd train hard for an upcoming competition. You'd prepare hard for an upcoming arts festival if you were a ballerina. How about you do the same for childbirth? Your body goes through many changes during pregnancy, and they may be as tough on you as any other sport.

As your belly grows to accommodate the baby, your center of gravity also shifts. This has been known to affect posture in pregnant women. If you are in a position to, find a physical therapist to help you train and reduce the chances of pains and injuries during pregnancy and birth. If not, you can join your local pregnant women's yoga and meditation or exercise classes. Alternatively, you can find exercises and tutors for pregnant women online and do them in the comfort of your home.

You will get exposure to helpful exercises that teach you how to push and get into different and comfortable positions during birth. What's more, practice and training strengthen your muscles to have enough flexibility for delivery. Exercise also helps reduce avoidable muscle pains and aches after childbirth.

Understand labor positions

The most common birth position is - lying on your back. You may be familiar with it from movies, books, blogs, and stories from people who've given birth before. You may not know that these positions put a lot of pressure on your pelvis and the nerves around it. Try and learn how to change positions during labor if you can. You can walk or lie on your side during labor.

Trying out different positions might be challenging, but it can help the baby descend, reduce the pressure on your pelvic area and help eliminate the need for medical intervention. You can try sitting up too. This way, the necessary blood supply to your pelvic region is maintained.

Practice these positions before the big day, so you are familiar with them and what you can do to ease childbirth.

Change your diet

Your doctor will mention that now is the time to put alcohol and cigarettes aside. Reduce caffeine and processed foods too. Instead, go for healthy, whole, fresh, homemade meals. Find a nutritious diet plan that nourishes the growing baby and gives you enough energy to cater to the baby's needs and your own nutritional needs, and lets you stack up enough energy for childbirth.

Ask your doctor to recommend the right supplements and vitamins for your needs. Your body works ten times as hard to support your baby's nutritional needs. It's therefore important to add safe vitamins and supplements so your baby can grow healthy.

Get a dental check-up now. Gum disease is bad for pregnancy and your baby's health.

Prepare yourself for labor pains.

You've heard wild stories about labor pains. Most of it is true because contractions that lead to childbirth are very uncomfortable. Fortunately, you can manage these contractions naturally and reduce the need for medication. Here are some tips for dealing with labor pain.

- Find a calm, comfortable space with extra space so you can move around. A rocking chair or a soft mattress to lie on can be soothing.

- Surround yourself with people who care. It can be a midwife, a friend, a family member, or a partner; make sure you are not going through it alone.

Having a support system around can be reassuring and helps you deal with the pain better.

- Learn about labor. Make sure you are well-informed about what you should expect in the delivery room. Ask your doctor everything about labor you are unsure about. Discuss your worries and concerns, so you aren't going into labor uninformed.

- Rhythmic breathing exercises can help you deal with labor pains. As you exhale while doing rhythmic breathing, you release tension from around the body, which can be calming.

- Relax your muscles with massages using oil between the contractions.

Buy functional maternity clothes.

The maternity landscape has changed over the years. You can wear a wide range of fashionable maternity clothes and still feel beautiful and classy. Buy comfortable support wear that fits your changing body. Some are so efficient that they help reduce pregnancy pains and aches.

Stress management techniques

You may be excited about being a mother, and you are probably looking forward to when you can finally hold that bundle of joy in your arms. The only problem is you have to deliver the baby first before you can hold it. The problem is you are scared mindless. You are not alone. Many women struggle with anxiety, fear of the unknown, and worry about what will happen in the delivery room. While many women worry about this, around 6-10% have a chronic fear of childbirth.

This fear can manifest itself in the form of panic and anxiety attacks, nightmares, shortness of breath, and concentration difficulties. Who wants to deal with all this on top of everything else? Fortunately, there is so much you can do to manage the stress and anxiety associated with pregnancy.

Don't fall for the hype.

It might look like everyone else is okay and doing well with their pregnancies. It might look like everyone else is having it easy, and you are the only one struggling. The truth is every pregnant mother faces their fair share of challenges. So many women admit that they struggle with mood swings and low spirits during pregnancy and after childbirth. The only problem is that some of them can hide it better than others, more so in public.

You are dealing with many hormones and might feel emotional at times – this is okay. It's important to understand your situation and talk to someone when you need to. If you realize that you feel sad more days than excited, it might be time to talk to someone.

Therapy is an option.

In a Finnish study on pregnant women who underwent therapy, experts discovered that the women had shorter labor periods and many avoided unnecessary C-sections. While many of the women in the study had an extreme fear of labor, therapy helped them deal with it, and they eventually had a more straightforward birth than those who didn't.

If your fear of childbirth takes over your life, so there is nothing else you can do except replay worse case scenarios in your head, a therapist might be the one thing you need. You may find reassurance by talking to someone who understands and has possibly gone through the same thing. You'll realize childbirth is a normal, natural part of life that doesn't have to be scary or upsetting.

Block out negativity

Don't feed on the negativity you see on TV, social media, or from friends and family. Some people have negative stories about childbirth, and while labor pains might be uncomfortable for every woman, it doesn't mean you'll have the same experience as them. You've been training, exercising, and learning what to expect during labor. You already know you can manage, and you'll give birth to a healthy baby.

While most people sharing stories with you online are genuinely concerned about your well-being and have the best intentions, others speak from the point of ignorance. Fear of childbirth has been made ten times worse by over-dramatization of delivery by people who want to get a reaction from others. Filter the noise and focus on positivity.

You can opt for pain relief.

Think about it for a minute, and you'll realize what scares you the most is the pain you anticipate during labor and childbirth. Maybe if you learned that there are many safe and effective options for relief, you could go into this a little confident. Medication is also an option if you are interested.

Talk to your healthcare provider about what's best for you and the child. Should you go for medication? Which options are safest, and what pain-relief methods are on the table? Which birth intention should you choose? After listening to their advice, you can decide the best way forward.

Stay active

I discussed training and exercise as a way to prepare yourself mentally for childbirth. It is excellent for your physical health during pregnancy too. When you exercise, your body releases the feel-good hormones that improve your spirits and mood. It doesn't have to be as hard as going to the gym every day or doing vigorous aerobics for hours.

You can stay active by walking a few miles every day. If you need to grab something light from a nearby grocery shop, you can leave the car home and walk to and from there instead. You'll feel good when you come back from the walk with a clear mind and a stress-free spirit. Regular exercise is good for the baby too.

Go online and find safe pregnancy exercises you can do during every trimester.

Have some "me time."

Take a day off or a few hours off to do something you love. Find something you enjoy that is all for you. You can soak in a bath, listen to some calming music, visit your favorite restaurant and eat your favorite meal, go on a walk, meet up with the girls or do something else you enjoy. Whatever makes you happy, take some time to do it alone without distractions.

If you'd rather not be alone, you can find a local group of pregnant women you can hang out with whenever you need someone who understands. You can also create a little club where all of you can feel a sense of belonging. These women might become the strong support system you need when you give birth eventually.

Take a break when you feel overwhelmed.

Pregnancy symptoms can overwhelm you sometimes. As much as you'd like to stay cheerful and excited, the constant fatigue, swollen feet, and discomfort associated with pregnancy may take its toll on you after some time. Take a break and rest as much as you need.

It would be best to be realistic about how much you can do during pregnancy. You might be scared to take some time off, fearing you'll disappoint someone or let them down. You might struggle with boundaries and the idea of saying no, but you must put yourself and the baby first. You need to take care of your physical, mental, and emotional health now more than ever. Remember, stress affects your baby, too, and this isn't something you want.

People who love and understand you will not be offended by you putting yourself first while you are pregnant.

Relaxation exercises will help you deal with labor and pregnancy

Relaxation exercises like meditation and self-hypnosis can calm you down when you feel anxious and overwhelmed during pregnancy. You can also use them to calm yourself down during labor.

To calm your anxious spirit, you can also listen to peaceful, relaxing podcasts, music, and guided tapes. You may be unaware, but cyclic stress can lead to premature birth because it rubs off on your baby. You don't want to put your baby through this even before being born.

Prenatal yoga has been proven to have calming effects on pregnant mothers. If you can find time between your doctor's appointments, "me-time," and time with friends and family to do some calming prenatal yoga routines, you'll improve your physical and mental health.

CHAPTER THREE

Preparing for Baby

Your life changes forever as soon as you find out you are pregnant. Now you have to plan not just for yourself but for your baby's arrival. You may find your head spinning as you think of everything you need to do before childbirth. Any parent's worst thing is to overlook an important step and complicate things on their big day.

Fortunately, pregnancy is nine months long, and you have a lot of time to prepare for the baby's arrival. You need to start as soon as the test returns positive so you are not overwhelmed when the baby is almost due. Try to get everything you need to do out of the way to prepare well for the special day when it arrives.

So, what should you do in preparation for the baby's arrival?

Find a trustworthy healthcare provider.

Everyone longs for a different birthing experience. Some want an intimate at home-delivery with the help of a midwife, others may choose an OBGYN if they are to have a C-section or they've had a difficult pregnancy. Both are okay; remember, everyone's pregnancy experiences and preferences are different. Whichever way, it's time to shop for a healthcare provider and let them lead the way.

If you have people around you, friends, family, or a support group, you may get recommendations from expert healthcare providers on what to look out for. It's crucial to find a healthcare provider with whom you have a connection. If you have any personal issues and problems, you'll be free to open up and ask for help.

Steps to take when choosing your healthcare provider

Referrals from friends and family or other doctors are mostly how pregnant women choose their healthcare provider. But how do you know if the recommended healthcare provider is the one? The answer to this question is subjective. It feels like a bit of a matchmaking thing, to be honest.

Remember, everyone's experience is different, and what works for someone may not work for you. Either way, the best place to start is to meet the doctor in person and see if you have a personal connection with them during your consultation.

First, does the doctor listen intently to your concerns? Do they address them carefully? Are they patient while talking to you, or are they in a hurry to get done with you and move along? While addressing your worries, did they use a language you understand, or were they throwing around medical jargon that you couldn't wrap your head around? Did their secretary pick it up immediately when you first got their contact? Did they follow up on your case? You have to ask yourself these questions and many others.

Once all these questions are answered, you can go deeper and think about how to:

Arrange a meeting with the healthcare provider and their team

You already have a due date in place, but by now, you know babies arrive when they want. It may be impractical to book the doctor for a specific date because this may cause re-scheduling problems if the baby doesn't arrive on the agreed date. Besides, doctors have lives too, and they may have other things or even other patients lined up for those new dates.

For these reasons, I would recommend familiarizing yourself with the team. Hence, if your favorite doctor is not available, you are no stranger to the people who'll take over and assist you in the delivery room. The truth is good doctors aren't that available. Keep this in mind and understand that the sooner you start, the better.

Does the doctor do scans and blood tests on site?

It's frustrating for a busy mother-to-be with so many places to be sent across town for some simple scans and blood tests.

The good news is that most OBGYNs do everything in their offices. You'll get checked, blood tests, and scans in the same place, so you don't need to worry about going back and forth.

It would be best to keep in mind that every clinic works differently. In some, you'll get a nurse practitioner to work with throughout your pregnancy unless you have a high-risk pregnancy. In others, your antenatal appointments will be split between nursing practitioners and the OBGYN from time to time or if the doctor is not available. Make sure you are okay with the arrangement at hand; if not, you may want to move along.

Is the neonatal unit on-site? Have you seen it?

Visit the neonatal unit and see if you are happy with the place. The hospital must have a well-equipped, satisfactory unit on site. There should be everything needed for birth in one place. This way, if any complications arise during and after birth, you'll be at ease knowing that your team will take good care of the baby.

You have to look for an experienced health care provider and a competent team in a hospital that is well-equipped with necessary resources.

Medical history

Your pregnancy may fall in the high-risk spectrum if you live with chronic illnesses like high blood pressure or diabetes. If you've had complications with previous pregnancies, you may want extra care. Get blood screening and tests for other conditions you may not know about.

Specialization in twin births and IVF pregnancies has been rising recently, so you'll find some healthcare providers who lean more towards that. Make sure to ask for recommendations if that's what you prefer.

Would you rather have a home birth?

There are many alternatives to having your child born under an obstetrician's care. General physicians and midwives can help you bring your baby into this world at home and in an intimate environment. This trend has been growing in the last decade or more. While home birth can have extraordinary experiences, especially when everything goes as planned, it's essential to put an emergency plan in place if anything happens during or after birth.

If you are planning a home delivery, make sure not to miss any of your appointments throughout your pregnancy. This way, if you need the help of an obstetrician in the event of an emergency, you aren't strangers meeting for the first time in a delivery room.

Keep in mind that labor is complicated, and you might end up in the hospital even if your best choice was a home delivery. You know what's best for you and the baby but always keep an open mind. Safety is the most important thing.

Check your health insurance coverage.

What's the extent of your insurance coverage? Does it cover things like your blood work and scans? Will you have to worry about prenatal care? Does the insurance cover outpatient appointments? If it doesn't, what's the plan? You'll need to find another way to go about the situation and figure out the best way forward.

If you need to make any changes to your health insurance coverage, today is the day to get it done. Make adjustments before the baby arrives. If you need to adjust your finances, you have to do that now. Ask for help if you need to. Just make sure there are no surprises when it's time to have the baby.

If employed, you'll have to think of the workplace policy and maternity leave.

Work policy and rules regarding maternity leave differ from one workplace to another. However, you may be protected against loss of work or wages when you have a baby by the Family and Medical Leave Act. Depending on the kind of employee you are, you may be entitled to either paid or unpaid leave and job protection. If you have a partner, they may get these privileges too.

Talk to your boss or superior about the available options early enough, so there are no misunderstandings later on. This way, you can prepare yourself mentally and fill out the necessary paperwork on time. You may compensate for those weeks with vacation and sick days later if you are lucky enough.

Outline the baby's checklist

It will be your baby's first day outside the protection of your womb. They are very delicate. You'll want to make sure everything on your baby's checklist is in perfect condition.

- Have their clothes/beddings been washed? Make sure to use chemical-free detergents just in case the baby is allergic.

- Have you stocked up on nappies? Are you planning to use disposable or reusable nappies? You can also visit local retail shops to see if any trial packs are offered.

- Have you chosen the outfit they'll go home in? This is usually a fun exercise for expectant mothers. Try doing this with your partner or a friend to see what you settle for.

- Is the nursery set up yet? Nurseries take a while to complete, so you'll want to start sooner. You'll need a changing table, baby bathtub, bedsheets, bassinet, blankets, etc.

- Don't forget baby clothes, wipes, bibs, etc.

- You'll need a car seat and bottles, among other things.

Make sure you don't forget to buy any essential items. Your support person can help you remember or shop around for baby stuff. You'll never get to do this again, at least not for this baby, so have fun while you are at it.

Hospital bag

As big and exciting as the birth-day is, you may feel overwhelmed trying to remember all you need for those first days with your baby at the hospital or birthing center. And don't forget about yourself – this is also a time for mamma to take care of herself.

It would be best if you kept everything organized by packing three separate bags:

1)   A small bag containing a change of clothes and everything you'll need throughout labor and delivery.

2)   A medium-sized bag containing infant necessities such as clothes, blankets, diapers, and skincare baby lotion.

3)   An overnight bag including everything you'll need throughout your stay at the hospital. Don't forget to bring a bag to put your dirty laundry in!

You'll want to carry everything you need. Since each hospital has different policies regarding what they can supply, it's better to be prepared.

At first, your baby will do nothing more than eat and sleep. All they need is love, food, and warmth. Although the hospital will give you lots of blankets to keep your baby warm, there are a few more items you should bring with you:

- Swaddles and blankets –The hospital will most likely have blankets available, although they are unlikely to be particularly comfortable. Pack some of your own to keep your baby warm and swaddled while out and about.

- Socks and hats to keep your new arrival warm.

- At least three burp cloths, as your infant will most likely spit up a lot.

- Nursing pillow to support the baby during breastfeeding.

- Baby wipes for yourself and the baby.

Birth plan

A birth plan is a set of written or oral instructions that you, your partner, and your birth attendants can follow during labor and delivery. It can help you communicate what kind of care you want during labor, delivery, and the newborn period.

Birth plans may include information about pain relief options and the number of visitors you want in the room. Your birth plan also includes other preferences for services such as bathing your baby, taking them home from the hospital, and using a pacifier or bottle.

Keep a copy of your birth plan with you at all times. The maternity team who will be caring for you during your labor will discuss it with you so that they are aware of your wishes.

There's no "right way" of writing a birth plan. You can do it on the fly by scribbling down a few of your main concerns and bringing them up with your practitioner during your next appointment.

Listen to what your doctor says about your labor alternatives once you've discussed your preferences regarding your childbirth experience. Update your birth plan if there are any adjustments you need to make.

You may want to include items like:

- Who you'd like to be your birth partner and where you'd like to give birth.

- The labor positions you prefer.

- The form of pain relief you would like to use during labor.

- The type of music you'd like to listen to while giving birth.

- How you'd like to deliver the placenta?

- Special facilities, such as a birthing pool.

- How you would like your baby to be fed after birth?

- Your preferences for skin-to-skin contact with your newborn and cord clamping delay.

Although there's a fair chance your plan will be carried out exactly as you wrote it, there's always the chance it won't, and you may need to modify your birth plan at the last minute. As a result, flexibility is the most critical aspect of a good birth plan. Childbirth is surprisingly unpredictable: Even the best-laid ideas don't always go as planned.

Baby-proofing your house

When babies start crawling, they become more aware of their environment. They'll want to explore and discover their surroundings. Unfortunately, this discovery period can be disastrous, and it can even result in tragic mishaps.

It may not feel like it right now, but learning to baby-proof your home is an awesome responsibility. You're officially in charge of another life's safety. It would be best if you did everything necessary to protect your rambunctious little goober from a life filled with bumps, bruises, and one too many trips to the doctor's office.

Apart from keeping your baby safe, baby-proofing comes with other benefits like:

- It gives you peace of mind.

Keeping an eye on your infant can be exhausting, especially if you're a first-time mother. Instead of rushing up and down the halls to keep your child safe, baby-proofing your home will address your child's safety issues.

- It saves you money- Your toddler is likely to break and ruin valuable items in your home as they crawl around. Baby-proofing your home can prevent such losses.

Here are some baby-proof materials you should consider:

- Doorknob covers secured with child-proof locks.

- TV and furniture straps.

- Safe-plate outlet covers.

- Cardinal Gates cord safety wraps.

- Retractable gate demands.

- Eco-baby magnetic safety locks.

- Baby-proofing table corner guards.

- Window stops.

- Placemats.

While baby-proofing your home ensures safety for your child, their activities spell out danger alerts, and it's important to have emergency plans in place.

Some emergency measures to put in place include:
- Learning first aid and CPR for newborns and children aged 12 months and up is essential.

- Get some first-aid items. Ensure babysitters and other caretakers are aware of the location of the first-aid kit in your home and how to respond in an emergency.

- Programming emergency numbers into your home and cell phones is a good idea. Keep a list of these phone numbers by each phone in your home and distribute it to all caregivers.

- Install a fire extinguisher on each floor of your home and have it maintained or checked as directed by the manufacturer.

Make arrangements for younger kids, if any.

Figuring out what your other kids will do while you're recovering after giving birth to their new sibling can be overwhelming. You'll need help from others with this. Involve your partner, a friend, or a family member.

Consider employing a babysitter to look after the younger children if your partner has a busy work schedule. It's also crucial to talk to your other children about the shift so that they are prepared. Make them aware that their little sibling will require extra attention, but mummy will always be there.

Ongoing baby expenses

You may have heard people (especially those who haven't had kids) say that babies don't cost very much—but how would they know?

Soon after giving birth, you'll realize that those little costs add up quickly. Newborn clothing, diapers, and feeding supplies like bottles and burp cloths can add hundreds of dollars to your annual baby budget. Here are some ongoing baby expenses to consider.

Babycare

The cost of child care varies depending on where you live, your child's age, how much care they need, and what sort of care you use. According to the Care Index, the cost of in-center child care is just under $10,000 per year.

The average cost of a nanny or other in-home care is roughly $28,350 per year. However, this might vary depending on geography and other factors. Keep in mind that some costs, such as the child and dependent care credit, may be offset by other tax credits. Always double-check to see if you're eligible.

Clothes

According to many experts, new parents should budget roughly $50 per month for their child's first clothing year. The fee varies widely depending on personal desire and financial constraints, but the lowest end of the spectrum is roughly $25 each month.

Diapers

Diapers vary in price, but experts recommend setting aside at least $75 per month for diapers. If you choose disposable diapers, you should anticipate using up to 3,000 diapers in your child's first year alone.

Food

You should anticipate spending around $50 each month after you start giving your child solid meals. Compared to what a teenager will spend on food, children's early food costs are pretty low.

Hospital visit

Children are a wonderful gift—albeit costly at times. Expect three to four wellness appointments for exams, vaccines, other routine procedures and a few additional visits if the child falls ill. Some costs should be covered by your health insurance policy.

For the most part, good health insurance can protect you against hospital expenditures, but only careful planning and budgeting can help you deal with the rest.

CHAPTER FOUR

Diet and Nutrition

What happens with poor nutrition during pregnancy?

When you are pregnant, your body needs more nutrients than before. It's no secret that the growing baby also needs nutrients. Studies show that babies born to malnourished mothers are more likely to suffer the crippling effects of malnutrition. How sad is it that the child of a malnourished mother is nine times more likely to die in its first year? It is extremely important to eat healthy foods for you and your baby whenever possible.

Poor nutrition is broadly classified into two; **malnutrition** and **micronutrient deficiency.**

Malnutrition occurs when you do not eat enough food; the energy required exceeds calorie intake. Lack of appetite during pregnancy can result from morning sickness symptoms such as vomiting and nausea, common during the first 12 weeks of pregnancy (first trimester).

Insufficient food intake is linked to retarded intrauterine development of the infant. The risks are high and may include disruption of the baby's neurological, cardiovascular, digestive, and respiratory systems development. The child's brain may be damaged, and most organs will be underdeveloped. An infant may die while still in the womb or die within seven days after birth if the birth weight is significantly low.

Micronutrient deficiency occurs when your diet lacks vital nutrients, such as calcium, iron, folic acid, and zinc. A poor-nutrient diet may lead to anemia, infection, high blood pressure, and excessive bleeding, which may cause maternal death. While poor socio-economic status is usually linked to micro-nutrient deficiency, some underlying conditions can precipitate it.

For example, say you're pregnant, have epilepsy, and are on anti-epileptic medications. Taking the average dose of folic acid daily (400-600mcg) won't be enough. The anti-epileptic medications lower folic acid levels. You'll need to increase the level of folic acid to cater to your baby's nutritional needs. Just make sure you take no more than 1mg per day to avoid cardiovascular diseases and stroke.

Taking insufficient amounts of folic acid during pregnancy may cause neural tube defects, which are abnormalities that affect the brain and spinal cord. Neural tube abnormalities can cause paralysis, incontinence, and intellectual incapacity.

Depending on the vitamin or mineral and the stage of pregnancy, you'll be expected to take different supplements for you and your baby's well-being. Some vitamins and minerals improve your baby's physical development; others help keep your body healthy.

Symptoms and conditions developed due to poor diet choice

Your baby's needs are high during pregnancy. They'll need sufficient nutrients and minerals intake, which you must offer. If you don't choose the proper diet while pregnant, their growth can be affected significantly. A poor diet negatively impacts your baby's health and may even cause early intervention in the pregnancy.

Preterm birth is directly linked to malnutrition and micronutrient deficiency in expectant mothers. Genetics aside, these two are the leading causes of children's developmental problems and lifelong disorders. Poor diet during pregnancy can weaken your baby's bones and heart, and increase the risk of chronic diseases.

Over the last ten years, the number of overweight and obese women has increased dramatically, directly impacting their babies' birth weight. Studies show that obese expectant mothers have higher blood sugar levels, which means their infants will be heavier at delivery and are more likely to become obese later in life. Obese mothers give birth to obese children, who are at a high risk of developing conditions like Blount's disease.

When a newborn is malnourished, nutrients are directed to the heart, brain, adrenal glands, and placenta, while other organs (such as the bones, pancreas, muscles, and lungs) suffer. When low-birth-weight newborns have periods of abundant nourishment later in childhood and adulthood, they are more likely to become obese.

Low birth weight is linked to a higher adult blood pressure and, as a result, an increased risk of heart disease. Underweight babies who gain weight quickly in the first 6-12 months of life ('catch up growth') are more likely to develop excess body fat later, putting them at risk for obesity. When the mother's diet is poor, the risk of diabetes in the child is high.

Organs, including the pancreas, do not develop as they should if a baby is malnourished during pregnancy. The pancreas produces insulin crucial for managing blood sugar levels by allowing cells to convert sugar to energy. The pancreas may generate less insulin if it has not grown normally, increasing the risk of diabetes.

According to a study published in the New England Journal of Medicine, poor dietary habits during pregnancy harm the growing hearts of unborn children. Heart disease is considerably more likely in babies who become overweight or obese later.

New findings suggest that some restrictive diets adopted by pregnant women can cause serious harm to the unborn child. Malnutrition and lack of vitamins in a woman's diet during pregnancy are directly linked to increased risk of contracting cancer by adults who were underweight newborns.

Poor diet during pregnancy can affect the intelligence of an unborn child. Low nutrient intake can lower your child's IQ by 5 points. If babies are born too tiny or too big for their gestational age or born prematurely, their brain anatomy and development may be harmed.

Healthy bacteria colonize our guts; they help prevent dangerous bacteria from proliferating, improve nutrient absorption and boost the immune system. Gut bacteria establish themselves during the birth process, milk feeding and weaning, and stabilize at two years. Low-birth-weight newborns and premature babies have fewer and less diverse bacteria in their stomachs.

Poor diet during pregnancy can affect the development of healthy gut bacteria in infants. For instance, if a mom has a high level of the most abundant gut bacteria-derived from meat and eggs but low levels of staphylococcus and bifidobacterium, her child will also suffer the same problem.

Vitamins and prenatal supplements

Start taking prenatal vitamins as soon as possible after conception. Taking a prenatal vitamin every day is recommended for women of reproductive age. Below is a list of some of the prenatal vitamins you should take while pregnant:

Zinc

It is essential for the fetus' early development, as it aids in the survival and growth of the fundamental organs required for future growth. A deficit at this time in the pregnancy can be fatal to your kid and may result in a miscarriage.

Zinc strengthens the immune system, aids wound healing, and synthesizes proteins and DNA. During pregnancy, 11mg of zinc per day will suffice.

Oysters are well-known for having the highest zinc content per serving of any food. Most people obtain their zinc from poultry and red meat.

However, if you consume a predominantly vegetarian diet, you may find it challenging to get enough zinc from food alone. Because plant foods are more difficult to absorb zinc from, supplements may help.

Calcium

Throughout the pregnancy, calcium aids in the proper growth of the fetus. It is the most critical mineral for the development of your baby's bone and skeletal systems. Calcium also helps with your baby's nerve development. Low calcium intake may lead to rickets and underdeveloped sensation and motor function.

If you don't take enough calcium during pregnancy, you may develop osteoporosis too.

You need to take about 1000mg of calcium a day during pregnancy.

Iron

You need to take about 27mg of iron per day during pregnancy, almost double the amount when not pregnant. Iron makes hemoglobin, a component of red blood cells that carries oxygen. It is essential for the normal development of your child's brain.

Lack of iron is synonymous with anemia. The lack of oxygen for the baby may damage brain cells, leading to death in-utero.

Meat, chicken, fish, beans, fortified cereals, and spinach are high in iron.

Vitamin B12

It helps synthesize DNA and prevents neural tube abnormalities. Chicken, eggs, beef, pork, and fish contain vitamin B12.

Vitamin B12 deficiency during pregnancy can harm your unborn baby's DNA synthesis. Vitamin B12 deficiency during pregnancy can lead to an underweight baby. It can also lead to metabolic abnormalities in the infant, such as Type 2 diabetes.

You will need at least 2.6mcg of vitamin B12 during pregnancy.

Omega-3

Taking omega-3 supplements throughout pregnancy helps keep your hormones in check. It reduces health problems caused by allergic reactions and inflammation.

Omega-3 fatty acids enhance your mood and help you avoid depression and the benefits listed above. During pregnancy, these disorders afflict a large number of women. Getting enough omega-3 in your diet can protect you from certain malignancies, such as breast cancer. It also keeps your blood pressure and kidneys in check.

Taking the correct doses of omega-3 throughout pregnancy aids with the development of your unborn baby's eyes and brain. Omega-3 also aids in the prevention of preterm labor. It helps get the baby to a normal birth weight, increases the amount of breast milk produced, and aids in the development of your baby's cognitive abilities.

Multiple studies report that consuming enough omega-3 protects your baby from allergies.

Fish, dark green vegetables, walnuts, sesame seeds, mustard seeds, sunflowers, and fortified foods such as eggs, juice, bread, and soybeans contain omega 3.

Omega-3 supplements are available in various formats, including liquid, gel, and chewable tablets. Some of them are flavored to disguise the taste of fish. Fish oil is used in the majority of omega-3 supplements.

Some omega-3 supplements are derived from algae or sea plants. These contain no mercury, have no fishy flavor, and are suitable for vegetarians.

When purchasing an omega-3 supplement, make sure the label says it has been filtered to remove PCB contamination. You should also make sure the supplement contains at least 200 mg of omega-3. Reduce your intake of processed and fried foods during pregnancy to optimize your body's utilization of omega-3.

Thiamine (vitamin B1)

Thiamine is vital during pregnancy because it helps develop your baby's brain and allows you and your baby to turn carbs into energy.

Thiamine can be found in fortified cereals, lean pork, and whole grains, among other foods. During pregnancy, 1.4mg of thiamine per day is enough.

Riboflavin (vitamin B2)

Vitamin B2 is necessary for energy production during pregnancy. Its advantages include increasing the baby's growth, maintaining good skin, and improving vision.

It can also aid in developing the baby's muscles and bones and alleviate various pregnancy symptoms such as exhaustion and nausea. You need 1.4mg of vitamin B2 per day during pregnancy.

Vitamin B6

Vitamin B6 is essential for your baby's developing brain and nerve system during pregnancy. It also aids your baby's protein and glucose metabolism.

You should be able to acquire all of the vitamin B6 you need from your diet and prenatal vitamins during pregnancy. According to some research, vitamin B6 can aid with morning sickness.

Vitamin E

It has antioxidant properties and reduces the chances of getting preeclampsia by decreasing oxidative stress.

Eicosapentaenoic acid (EPA) and docosahexaenoic acid (DHA) are two types of fatty acids. These fatty acids are essential for embryonic brain development so you will need more of them throughout pregnancy. Some prenatals include them, but the majority don't. Most pregnant women take supplemental DHA and EPA, such as fish oil or algal oil.

Other essential vitamins and minerals included in prenatal supplements are; niacin, biotin, pantothenic acid, choline, iodine, magnesium, selenium, copper, manganese, chromium, molybdenum, potassium, inositol, betaine HCL, and vitamins A, C, D3, and K.

Food safety guidelines

Being pregnant can be an exciting time, but you have to take special care to ensure your baby stays safe and healthy. Your immunity is at its weakest during pregnancy, increasing your chances of developing foodborne illnesses. Even one infection can be life-threatening to the fetus, leading to a miscarriage or other serious medical complications such as preterm delivery or stillbirth. Knowing what foods are safe and how to store them properly will help prevent infection.

If you can't cook your food, purchase cooked and ready-to-eat foods that have been properly stored and reheated. When buying grilled foods from restaurants, ask about the food safety inspection procedures of the business.

Listeriosis, salmonellosis, and toxoplasmosis are the three most serious food borne infections for pregnant women.

Listeriosis

Listeria monocytogenes is a bacteria prevalent in water and soil. The bacteria causes listeriosis. It is present in processed meals like cheeses and cold cuts, vegetables, meats, and dairy products. Although listeria bacteria pose minimal risk to a healthy person, they can cause early labor, serious infection in the baby, or even death of the fetus while still in the womb.

To avoid getting listeriosis, reheat hot dogs, deli meats, and luncheon meats before eating. Don't eat blue-veined, feta, camembert, brie, and Mexican cheeses like "queso Blanco fresco."

Avoid drinking unpasteurized milk and eating meals that contain it. Don't consume store-bought salads like ham, tuna, chicken, seafood, or eggs.

Toxoplasmosis

Toxoplasma gondii parasite is the culprit associated with toxoplasmosis. Toxoplasmosis can be transmitted to a fetus by a pregnant woman. Stillbirth, miscarriage, and congenital abnormalities are possible outcomes of fetal toxoplasmosis. The parasite enters the body when you swallow the eggs of toxoplasma gondii from the soil or contaminated surfaces. Clean your hands thoroughly after cleaning a cat's litter box, gardening, or touching dirt.

Follow these measures to avoid contracting toxoplasmosis:

• All foods, including commercial fruits and vegetables, that may have been exposed to cat feces should be washed.

• Avoid dried meats and consume previously frozen or well-cooked meat only. To kill toxoplasma gondii, cook meat using high temperatures or expose it to extremely low temperatures.

• Wash your hands and utensils thoroughly after preparing seafood, poultry, fruits, raw meat, or vegetables.

• Avoid drinking untreated water.

• Keep cat waste out of the house and out of the garden.

Salmonellosis

Frequent food infection is caused by eating foods contaminated with salmonella bacteria. Animals, including humans, spread the bacteria when they come into indirect or direct contact with them. Salmonella don't thrive in the freezer or refrigerator, and heating your food above 73 degrees Celsius kills them.

Follow these recommendations to avoid getting salmonellosis:

• Practice standard hygiene procedures such as washing hands with warm water and soap, particularly after using the washroom and before handling food.

• Wash your hands and work surfaces thoroughly after handling raw meat, poultry, or fish.

• Take your time to rinse vegetables and fruits before consumption.

Foods to avoid while pregnant

We all have our favorite foods. Some of us eat them every day. But what about when you are pregnant? Are the foods you are eating healthy for your baby? Think before you bite into that cheeseburger or order that box of pizza and fries!

The foods on this list should be avoided during pregnancy, as they contain high amounts of toxins that may hurt the baby.

The list below shows foods to avoid when pregnant:

• **Processed meats**

DO NOT EAT unless it's been wholly cooked to at least 75 degrees Celsius and should be eaten right away.

- **Raw meat**

DO NOT EAT. Purchase freshly prepared food and consume it while it is still hot.   Refrigerate leftovers and reheat to at least 60°C within a day.

- **Poultry**

Ensure the chicken is adequately cooked, at least 74 degrees Celsius, and eat it while still hot. Any leftovers should be kept in the fridge and reheated to at least 60°C within a day.

- **Paté**

DO NOT EAT.

- **Seafood**

Cook to a minimum temperature of 63°C before serving. Reheat leftovers to at least 60°C in the refrigerator and consume within one day of cooking.

- **Sushi**

Don't eat raw meat or seafood; however if fully cooked eat it right away while hot.

111

- **Cooked meats**

Cook to a temperature of at least 71°C (medium) and serve immediately.

- **Cheese**

DO NOT EAT unless it's been wholly cooked to at least 75 degrees Celsius and eaten right away. Refrigerate and consume within two days of opening the package.

- **Ice-cream**

Frozen foods should be kept in the refrigerator.

- **Dairy**

Check the 'use-by' or 'best before date. Observe the storage instructions.

- **Custard**

If you opened it recently, you could eat it cold. Refrigerate to reheat to at least 60 degrees Celsius and use within one day of opening. Check the 'best before' or 'use-by' date on the product. Cook to a temperature of at least 71°C and serve immediately. Keep refrigerated. Reheat to at least 60°C and use within one day of preparation.

• Eggs

Cook to a temperature of at least 71°C. Use only fresh eggs that aren't broken or soiled.

• Salads

Before preparing and eating salads, thoroughly wash all salad ingredients; store any leftover salads in the refrigerator and use them within a day of preparation.

• Fruit

Wash thoroughly before eating.

• Vegetables

Before consuming raw or before cooking, wash thoroughly.

• Bean sprouts

DO NOT EAT raw.

- **Leftovers**

Refrigerate leftovers. Make sure they are covered while in the fridge. Reheat at 60°C before eating.

- **Canned foods**

Use any leftovers within a day by storing them in clean, sealed containers in the fridge.

- **Stuffing**

DO NOT EAT unless it has been cooked separately and is served hot.

- **Hummus & other dips containing Tahini**

DO NOT EAT.

- **Soy**

Check the 'use-by' or 'best before date. Observe the storage instructions.

- **Cold cuts and Deli Meat Sandwiches**

DO NOT EAT.

CHAPTER FIVE

Fitness and Exercise

The importance of exercise during pregnancy

Pregnancy can be exhausting, and to add to that, you may be very self-conscious about how your body has changed. While it is essential to take care of and listen to your body, exercise is vital for you and your baby. Exercises help your body prepare for the demands of pregnancy and childbirth and also increase your energy levels during this period.

Prenatal exercise benefits both the mother and baby and has long-term health effects that last a lifetime.

Benefits for the mother:

Regular exercise can help you stay fit during pregnancy and cope better with labor. Exercising makes it easier to regain your fitness following your child's birth.

You may have difficulty sleeping through the night as your pregnancy progresses. Regular physical activity will help you get a good night's sleep.

Exercise improves your posture and your mood. Hormonal changes during pregnancy might cause mood swings and make you feel stressed. Exercising every day helps to keep stress at bay. Interacting with other pregnant women during your fitness sessions can also be a terrific stress reliever.

Exercise decreases backaches, constipation, bloating, and swelling of the legs. It also improves your muscle tone, strength, and endurance and helps your body cope with pains and aches. Walking, stretching, and yoga are light workouts that can help relieve back pain, strengthen abdominal muscles, and increase blood circulation.

It increases your energy levels and may help prevent or manage gestational diabetes. It also aids in the control of blood sugar levels.

Morning sickness becomes less common as you exercise more. Pregnant women experience morning sickness in various ways ranging from extreme or only minor nausea. Exercise has been reported to minimize nausea and vomiting during pregnancy.

Exercise accelerates postpartum healing. If you stay inactive throughout pregnancy, it will be more challenging to go back into a regular fitness routine once your kid arrives. But if you stay active during pregnancy, you will get back on your feet faster after your baby is born.

Exercise reduces the risk of injury. Back and shoulder problems are among the most common complaints among women who have just given birth. While your kid may only weigh a few kilograms, pulling them in and out of the cot may cause back problems. Back exercises and strengthening will help you avoid injury.

Benefits for the baby

1)   **Prenatal exercise improves your baby's long-term health.**

Exercise during pregnancy may lower your baby's risk of getting juvenile diabetes and neonatal macrosomia, a condition in which babies are born abnormally large. Keep these healthy practices after the baby is born to teach them how to live a healthy lifestyle!

2) Exercises may improve your child's intelligence.

Studies show that children whose mothers exercised while pregnant have stronger memories and score higher on IQ and language exams.

Women who exercise throughout pregnancy have faster growing and functioning placentas than those who are healthy but don't exercise.

A study from the University of Montreal discovered that infants of active mothers showed brain activity like that of a mature brain. The brains of newborns born to mothers who exercised developed faster than those born to mothers who were more sedentary.

3) It prepares the baby for a smooth transition into the new world

According to research, newborns whose moms exercised throughout pregnancy can cope with labor pressures, such as contractions, better than kids whose mothers were inactive.

Studies show that kids whose mothers exercised can better adjust to life outside the uterus and are more attentive and easy to care for.

Exercise limitations

When is exercise too much during pregnancy?

Although women are generally encouraged to exercise during pregnancy, it's also important that you listen to your body and sense the amount of physical activity that feels right for you.

As a general guideline for exercising during pregnancy: talk with your doctor before starting a physical activity or exercise program, even if it's something you've done in the past. Pregnancy changes your body and needs, and your doctor has the best advice for your situation.

Start carefully and increase your activity gradually if you are new to exercising. You can start small, with as little as 5 minutes every day. Increase your activity by 5 minutes per week until you can stay active for 30 minutes per day.

If you were active before becoming pregnant, you might continue doing so with your doctor's permission. However, if you start losing weight, you may need to increase your calorie intake.

Aim for at least 150 minutes of moderate-intensity aerobic activity each week. Aerobic exercises help you work major muscles in your body in a rhythmic manner (such as those in your legs and arms). You're moving enough to get your heart rate up and sweating at a moderate effort.

Certain precautions apply when exercising during pregnancy:

- Drink lots of water before, during, and after your workout. Dizziness, a fast-pounding heart, and peeing small amounts of dark yellow urine are all signs of dehydration.

- To protect your breasts, choose a sports bra with a lot of support. A belly support belt can help you walk or run comfortably.

- Avoid exercises that make your body overheat, especially in the first trimester. Drink lots of fluids, dress comfortably, and exercise in a temperature-controlled environment. Don't exercise when it's extremely hot or humid outside.

Basic exercise routines during pregnancy and how to do them

By the time you're in your second trimester, you may feel more energetic and ready to exercise. But it's important to stick to safe workouts and exercise routines during pregnancy.

Having a baby is an amazing experience, but it does present some unique physical challenges. During pregnancy, you're probably wondering how to stay in shape and—more importantly—how to stay healthy.

As the baby grows at an incredible rate, your body constantly changes to accommodate the new life inside you. Your muscles stretch and become more flexible, sometimes making it harder for you to do things like bending over or lifting items.

Whether you are new to working out or are keeping up with a routine before the baby arrives, it is essential not to forget about your physical needs and health during pregnancy. During this time, your body needs more support than ever before, so it's in your best interest to keep moving as much as possible.

The exercises discussed below strengthen muscles, help with weight loss and reduce the risk of complications for you and your baby. They improve your posture and relieve common pregnancy symptoms like carpal tunnel syndrome and sciatica.

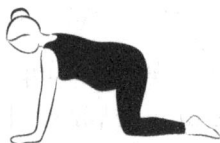

1)   4-point kneeling
This exercise strengthens abdominal muscles.
- Kneel on your hands and knees.

- Your hips should be directly over your knees, and your shoulders should be directly over your hands. You should have a straight back.

- Take a deep breath and exhale.

- Pull your abdominal muscles in as you exhale. This is what it means to engage your abdominal muscles.

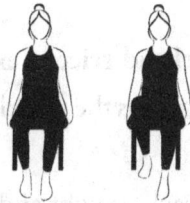

2) Sitting knee lift

This exercise strengthens your core muscles.

- Sit near the edge of a chair.

- Put your feet flat on the floor and flex your knees.

- Keep your hands under your thighs, with the palms facing down.

- Slowly bring your flexed knee toward your chest.

- Lower the leg and repeat with the contralateral leg.

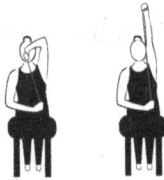

3)   Seated overhead triceps extension

This exercise strengthens the muscles at the back of your arms.

- Keep your back straight and your feet flat on the floor when seated.

- Raise your right arm and bend it at the elbow while holding a resistance band in the right hand. Reach behind your back with your left hand and grasp the resistance band's opposite end at the back of your waist.

- Raise and lower your right arm by flexing and extending your elbow close to your head. Keep the resistance band's opposite end fixed behind your waist.

- Repeat the process using the left arm.

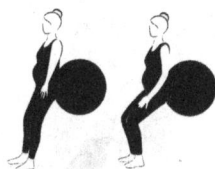

4)   Ball wall squat

It stretches the gluteus muscles and muscles of the leg. If you feel pain when performing this exercise, stop.

- Put the exercise ball close to the wall.

- Using your lower back, press the ball hard against the wall.

- Make sure your weight is evenly distributed between both feet.

- Squat down while firmly pressing against the ball with a slow, controlled movement.

- Keep your knees from collapsing inward.

- Keep your feet flat on the ground.

- Keep your chest open and your shoulders from rounding.

- If you can't squat down, start with half-squats.

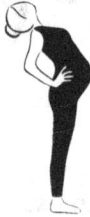

5)   **Standing backbend**

This exercise straightens the back and stretches the chest muscles.

- Place your palms at the back of each hip as you stand.

- Bend back around 15 to 20 degrees slowly.

- Hold the position for 20 seconds.

- Repeat 8 to 12 times.

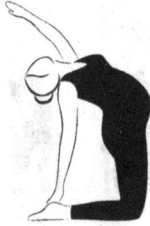

6)   Heel touch kneeling

It strengthens the muscles of the back and abdomen.

- Kneel on a workout mat.

- Rotate your body to the right in a calm, controlled motion.

- Touch your left heel with your right hand.

- For balance, extend your left arm above your head.

- Repeat the process on the other side.

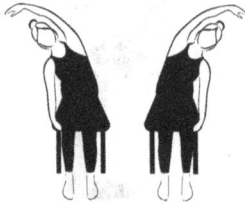

7)   Seated side stretch

It releases tension at the sides of your body.

- Sit up straight in a chair, maintaining your back neutral and your abdomen pushed in.

- Your feet should be flat on the floor, and your hips should be about as wide as your feet.

- Place your left hand on the back of your right knee.

- Raise your right arm and bend it to the left until a slight strain is felt.

- Breathe normally, don't slouch or stoop your shoulders, and hold the position for a few seconds.

- Repeat the process on the other side.

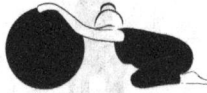

8) Ball shoulder stretch

Stretches the back, shoulder, and arms.

- Kneel with the exercise ball in front of you on the floor and place your hands on either side of the ball.

- Roll the ball while moving your buttocks back.

- Keep your gaze fixed on the ground.

- Make sure your neck isn't arched.

- To feel a gentle stretch, go only as far as is comfortable.

- Hold the position for a few seconds.

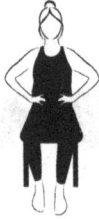

9) Core breath

This is one of the easiest abdominal exercises.

- Sit comfortably and straighten your back.

- Both hands should be on your waist.

- Inhale deeply, moving your chest outward, then exhale.

- Repeat eight to twelve times.

Staying active

During pregnancy, your body goes through many physical changes that can make you feel more tired than usual. You may be more aware of body aches and pains, but staying active can help you feel comfortable and connected with your baby. It may shorten your labor and speed up your recovery.

Being active can help you stay fit, improve your mood, and boost your energy level. Exercise can help you sleep better while you're pregnant. You will need as much sleep as you can get throughout this time.

It will be simpler to lose weight after delivery if you have a regular exercise plan. Enjoying a variety of pleasurable physical activities during pregnancy gives you the chance to have fun while helping your body stay strong and healthy. Staying active helps release endorphins, which can help keep you in a good mood, feeling fit and happy.

Being active during pregnancy may also reduce your risk of diseases such as diabetes (gestational diabetes), preeclampsia (high blood pressure at 20 weeks of pregnancy), and depression after giving birth (postpartum depression). Pay attention to your body and figure out what works best for you. Also, bear in mind that physical activity may feel different when pregnant. Try something else if an activity doesn't feel right.

Start by taking a walk in your neighborhood or at the mall. Inviting your partner and children to join you is a great idea. As it gets easier, increase the distance you walk each time. You can also perform low-grade activities, such as fitness walking, low impact dancing, swimming, recumbent bicycling, low step aerobics, or leaf raking. If you haven't been physically active before, start cautiously and gradually build up.

If your gym or community center offers a yoga class for pregnant women, inquire about it. You'll get to exercise and make some new friends also. Look for workout videos for pregnant moms online or borrow DVDs from the library to exercise on your own time and for free.

Consider walking instead of taking the bus. Instead of taking the elevator, take the steps. Stair climbing is an excellent way to tone your leg and abdominal muscles. Consider exiting the lift a few floors early if you are on an exceptionally high floor.

It is safe and recommended to continue lifting weights or perform other muscle-strengthening activities while pregnant. Remember that lifting weights is not the only technique to build muscle; you can also use resistance bands or perform body-weight exercises like squats and lunges. While doing muscle-strengthening exercises, make sure you're not holding your breath.

Above all, your safety and that of your child come first. After the first trimester (12 weeks of pregnancy), avoid activities that would have you lying flat on your back because they can disrupt blood flow to the fetus; instead, prop yourself up with a pillow. Avoid sports like downhill skiing or horseback riding that increase your chance of falling. Avoid activities like basketball or soccer where you could get smacked in the stomach.

Exercise to avoid during pregnancy

Ah, pregnancy. A time to quit worrying about yourself and start worrying about your offspring. Not all exercises are safe during pregnancy, though. Sometimes it can be hard to know which types of exercise are safe and which ones are not.

While it is essential to stay active during this period, safety should be your main priority. It is crucial to avoid exercises that could harm your growing baby or injure you.

The ten exercises you should avoid are:

1)   Sports that increase your chances of falling.

They include gymnastics, snowboarding, downhill skiing, vigorous racket sports (don't play singles; play doubles, instead), ice skating, outdoor cycling, horseback riding, diving, and contact sports (like ice hockey, basketball, or soccer), rollerblading, and bungee jumping.

2) Exercises that involve lying fully supine.

After the fourth month, you must avoid exercises that require you to lie flat facing up for long periods. The weight of your growing uterus may compress major blood vessels, restricting circulation for you and your baby. As a result, you may feel queasy, dizzy, and out of breath.

3) Hot yoga

Avoid any activity or setting that raises your body temperature above 37.5 degrees Celsius. Hot temperatures may cause dilation of blood vessels to the skin and away from the uterus to cool you down.

Avoid saunas, steam rooms, and hot pools. Hot yoga may lead to preterm labor and congenital abnormalities.

4) Exercises that build up abdominal pressure

Excessive pressure on the belly can cause a drop in blood pressure. For this reason, you must avoid exercises that put pressure on your abdominal area. Avoid abdominal crunches and knee bends, double leg raises, straight-leg toe touches, complete sit-ups, jarring actions, rapid changes in direction, bicycling, surfing, snowboarding, and waist twisting motions when standing.

Some alternative workouts to develop your abdominal muscles include squats, side rises, pilates, and Kegels.

5) Heavy weight lifting

Your tendons and ligaments become flexible since your body releases the relaxin hormone during pregnancy. Your center of gravity also changes as your bump becomes bigger.

Lifting heavy weights at this point could make you fall due to a shifted center of gravity. You may end up spraining your joints too.

6) Scuba diving

Don't scuba dive when pregnant. Air pressure rises as you plunge further into the water, and it is hazardous to you and your baby.

7) Aerobic exercises

Although moderate exercise is beneficial, avoid strenuous aerobic activities during the second or third trimester, especially if you have a cardiac condition, severe anemia, or chronic bleeding.

8) Boot camps

Most boot camps comprise pushing tires, using ropes, boxing, or lifting heavy weights, which can be dangerous to you and your baby.

Boot camps are meant for a healthy population. It's best if you don't get involved in boot camps during this time.

9) Exercises that will require you to hold your breath for an extended period.

Deep breathing exercises must be practiced during pregnancy. It promotes better blood and oxygen flow to the fetus, resulting in appropriate functioning and agility. Suppose you try to hold your breath for an extended period. In that case, your oxygen supply will be compromised, resulting in dizziness and breathlessness and a deficit of oxygen for your baby, which is extremely dangerous. So please take a deep breath and don't hold it for too long.

10) Exercises You've Never Done Before

If you are new to exercise, it's best not to do it because it could put your body under stress. Also, if you have never exercised before, start with the low-impact exercises and never do anything complicated after you've conceived. Start with mild workouts like walking or aqua-aerobics, which can help you burn calories while still being soft on your joints.

Warning signs you should not ignore during exercises

Being pregnant is a wonderful thing! There's so much to enjoy, including exercising. However, here are some red flags to look out for when exercising:

- Headache and chest pain.

- A quick heartbeat that isn't like what you're used to when exercising.

- Dizziness.

- Clear fluid or blood gushing from your vagina.

- Calf discomfort or swelling.

- Shortness of breath that isn't like what you'd get from exercising.

- Muscle weakness and fetal movement alterations.

- Discomfort in the hips, pelvis, or abdomen.

Stop what you are doing if you notice any of these signs. After taking a break, certain warning indicators, like dizziness and muscle weakness, may go away.

CHAPTER SIX

Mindfulness & Meditation

Pregnancy should be exciting, but many women are consumed by anxiety and fear of the inevitable physical pain of labor and childbirth. Sometimes, emotions overwhelm you unexpectedly; other times, the emotions creep up on you slowly. As the days go by, you notice that your relationships and work are affected by your wild, spiraling thoughts. How can you quiet the chatter in your head to enjoy your pregnancy?

Meditation and mindfulness can help you cope.

Studies show that mindfulness and meditation can help ease anxiety during pregnancy, especially in first-time mothers. It can also help them cope with fears of labor and childbirth. According to the BMC Pregnancy and Childbirth journal, mindfulness and meditation could help alleviate prenatal and postpartum depression and its symptoms in expectant mothers.

Other studies document benefits such as the birth of healthier babies with little to no developmental issues and improved spirits in women who practice mindfulness and meditation during pregnancy.

What is mindfulness about?

Mindfulness is about living in the moment – think about this moment, right here, right now. Stop worrying about the future and creating what-if scenarios that don't exist.

Be an open-minded individual – pregnant mothers don't always have that "pregnancy glow" throughout the 40 weeks. They worry during the night and deal with recurring pregnancy symptoms and everything they should be doing during the day. 18% of them are depressed, according to one study, and another 21% might be dealing with chronic anxiety.

Keep an open mind and practice mindfulness and meditation throughout pregnancy. Don't be too hard on yourself, and don't judge yourself for what you feel.

Compassion – You will make mistakes, and you will be imperfect. There is a high chance that you will carry on the attitude you adopt during pregnancy to parenthood. Have some self-compassion. This is a difficult journey, and you don't have to make it harder by being insensitive to yourself and your baby.

Steps to practice mindfulness during pregnancy

You don't have to spend hours on mindfulness and meditation to enjoy its benefits. You can carve a little time out of your busy schedule to practice simple mindful techniques, including those discussed below.

Mindful meditation

- Find a peaceful, quiet place with no interruptions.

- Sit and close your eyes.

- Focus on your breathing.

- Start by breathing slowly through your nose four times.

- Breathe out slowly through your mouth four times.

- All your attention should be on your breathing.

- Some thoughts will creep into your mind – don't fight them.

- Don't engage the thought; let it quickly pass through your mind.

- If you engage it and get lost in it for a while, that's okay. It's normal.

- Stop for a minute and turn your attention back to where you started.

The goal of this exercise isn't to get rid of the thoughts in your mind. Instead, this exercise helps you learn the simple art of awareness – being aware of your thoughts. Mindful meditation is about focusing on your thoughts and learning to live in the present moment, even with life's many interruptions.

As simple as they may look, these exercises may take a little while to master. Start slow with 1-, 2-, or 3-minute sessions once or twice a week. You can move on to longer 5-, 10-, or 15-minute sessions as you improve your mindfulness and meditation skills.

Use the steps described above to guide your meditation exercises, but you shouldn't limit yourself. There are multiple variations to the standard mindfulness practices you are familiar with. Find something that works for you and incorporate things you like into your routine.

You can try:

Music – If you can't find a quiet environment, you may appreciate some quiet music that you can focus on. Try meditation, yoga, or relaxing music that doesn't clutter the mind.

Fixate on your senses – what is happening around you? What can you feel, see or hear? It can be the sound of traffic, birds chirping, or wind blowing. Rest your hand on your lap and focus on other senses. What do you feel?

Using a candle - A candle gives you something to focus on, and many people love that. Find a quiet room and light a candle. Sit quietly and turn your focus on the flame, your thoughts, and the present moment.

It's also important to find a specific place to practice mindful meditation. It could be in a specific room in your house, on the beach, or in nature. Just make sure the place is calming and works for you.

If you struggle with this kind of meditation, you can try some guided meditations. Start by following a quick 2- or 3-minute guided meditation. Start by using guided meditation videos on YouTube or other meditation apps.

Yoga

If you can't sit still for extended periods, mindful yoga might be for you. You can incorporate mindfulness into your regular yoga practices. Try evaluating your senses while doing your yoga poses. Pay attention to what you think, feel, and hear. Strike a pose and concentrate on how it makes you feel.

Come back to the present moment. Focus on the thoughts that come with every yoga pose.

If you've never done yoga, you can find helpful yoga videos for pregnant women online.

Walking

Yes, you can practice mindfulness while you are walking. Focus on your thoughts, senses, and feelings as you walk. It doesn't matter where you are, whether in nature or walking down a busy road. Listen to the sounds and noises around you. Pay attention to what you see and hear.

Alternatively, you can narrow your focus to some specific thoughts. If you are walking down the street, you can focus on the gardens along your path. Stay in the present moment, and focus your thoughts on what you see in front of you.

Deep belly breathing

Breathing into your belly calms your nervous system, helping you relax and reduce overall stress. Belly exercises can help you bond with your baby too.

- Start by placing your hands on your belly. You can place one hand on your belly and one below your belly.

- Breathe in and out slowly but deeply.

- Focus on how this exercise makes you feel.

- Focus on how your belly rises and falls with every breath you inhale and exhale.

- You can start with a few minutes and add to them progressively if you've never done this before.

- Remember that you must be careful with breathing exercises and any other exercises. Don't hold your breath too long or breathe too fast. You don't want to do extreme exercises that can limit your baby's oxygen supply.

Exercises

Incorporate meditation into your exercise routine. Pay close attention to everything you feel with your movements. How do you feel when your feet hit the ground when running? How does it feel being outside? Is there something specific you hear? Your mind might wander from what you are doing; that's okay, but try your best to bring it back and focus on the task at hand.

Mantras

Words are powerful. Speak powerful words into your life and that of your baby. When you speak, you believe it easily. Words affect your subconscious, who you are, and your nervous system. You can say simple but powerful mantras as you exercise or do anything else.

For example:
- *You are a strong mother*

- *Breathe in for your baby*

- *You can do this for yourself and the baby*

- *Your baby needs this, etc.*

These mantras will also be helpful during labor and childbirth, so it's best to start practicing them now.

Practice mindfulness while doing everyday activities

You can practice mindfulness while doing almost anything; you don't need many hours if you don't have it. You can practice mindfulness and meditation while doing everyday tasks. Take on a mindful approach when doing anything and focus on the present moment entirely. Analyze your emotions and senses. If it's a physical activity, how does it make you feel? How does it sound?

For example, If you are brushing your teeth, you can focus on how the bristles feel on your teeth. How does the toothpaste taste in your mouth? How do the bristles sound as you are brushing your teeth?

If you're in a queue for something, and there are people around you, can you hear any sounds? Are the people around you talking? Is there movement around you?

If you are sitting at the office, can you hear people typing or the rustling of papers? Are some people walking past you? You can focus on how the chair you are sitting on feels or the smell of things around you.

Have a daily goal. You can take a break from everything you are doing at least twice a day to practice mindfulness.

Practice mindful fetal heartbeat awareness

You can use a fetal doppler to hear your baby's heartbeat before birth. Fetal dopplers are handheld gadgets that anyone can use. Being mindful of your baby's heartbeat while still in the womb can give you peace and joy.

- Start by spreading some ultrasound gel on your belly.

- Place the fetal doppler over the gel and move it around your belly until you hear your baby's heartbeat.

- Focus on the sound of the heartbeat over your headphones or speaker. Take a minute to appreciate the little heartbeat inside you. How does it make you feel?

- If your thoughts wander off, try to come back to the present moment and focus on the little heartbeat.

Mindfulness tips to follow

You can practice many mindfulness exercises during pregnancy, but you must do them right if you want them to be effective.

Start slowly but steadily.

Be gentle as you start your mindfulness and meditation exercises. Don't be too eager or go in with high expectations. Start slow and work steadily towards adding more minutes or hours if you like. You don't have to start by meditating or practicing mindfulness for hours; start with a few minutes, maybe 1 or 2 minutes, and increase the minutes gradually.

Once you are comfortable with the exercise you chose, you can set aside more time for it.

It may look or sound easy, but effective mindfulness is a skill that takes time to perfect. If you build the habit gradually, you will perfect it quickly, but if you are hasty, you may overwhelm yourself and never enjoy its benefits.

If you've identified an exercise you like, hold on to it. Add it to your daily mindfulness and meditation routine.

If you decide that you want to do 15-minute sessions, you can break them into 3 to 5-minute sessions throughout the day to improve effectiveness and blend them seamlessly into your daily routine.

Find something you can incorporate into your busy schedule

You have a lot to do, from doctors' appointments to shopping for baby items. Fortunately, there is at least one meditation exercise you can incorporate into your busy schedule. You don't have to go all-in either. As I said, don't be too hard on yourself.

Be mindful of your senses to and from work, on your morning jog, or as you drive to the doctor's office. If you can practice mindfulness while you do everyday activities, setting apart a specific time to do it will be unnecessary, especially if you are too busy.

You can still practice mindfulness after childbirth

Mindfulness and meditation have many benefits. While your life will change significantly once the baby arrives, you don't have to drop this habit altogether. You can create quick, short time frames to meditate when the baby is sleeping.

Try incorporating the practice into routine tasks such as breastfeeding or changing the baby.

Try mindfulness books

If you still have trouble getting used to mindfulness, you can read books to grasp the idea better. Try reading books about the relationship between mindfulness and pregnancy. Maybe you'll understand its importance better by reading.

Apps

You can download meditation apps if you want to do guided meditation.

There are so many meditation apps you can find online. Choose one that works for you. There are also guided meditation apps that are pregnancy-specific.

Classes

Look for mindfulness and meditation classes around your local area. You can also enroll in mindfulness and meditation classes as part of childbirth education classes.

Take control of your thoughts

You were thrilled when you first saw the positive pregnancy test, but 40 weeks is a long time, and you find yourself worrying about things that could go wrong frequently. Sometimes, these thoughts are too strong; you can't shake them off. Now it's affecting your life and your relationships. Besides, stress isn't good for the baby, so what can you do to take control of these thoughts?

Talk about what you feel and think.

Tell someone what you are worried about. If you have a partner, let them know. If not, talk to a friend, family member, or healthcare provider about your worries. They might offer you the support you need right now. Talking might be the "therapy" you need to keep negativity at bay.

If it's too much, you can ask your doctor to recommend a trustworthy therapist or a pregnant women specialist.

Find a hobby

Find something that helps lower your stress and anxiety. A good place to start would be physical activity. Engaging in physical activities leads to endorphin production – the body's feel-good hormone. Endorphins are like natural painkillers.

Try simple exercises like yoga, jogging, or walking. You don't have to do any of these things if you don't like them. Find something you enjoy. If it's dancing, do it. If it's aerobics, do it; make sure you get some slight movement from whatever you do.

Rest

Movement is good for you and the baby, but rest is also good. Get enough sleep and rest. You may struggle with sleep during pregnancy, especially in the second and third trimesters, but it could help with your anxiety if you can get enough rest.

If you don't sleep well during the night, try sneaking a few naps into your day.

Create a journal

Writing is an excellent way to express yourself, especially when you don't feel like talking. Don't just bottle your thoughts in; you'll overwhelm yourself. Pour your thoughts down on paper. Write everything you feel in a journal and express yourself without fear.

Creating a journal will also help you organize your thoughts, worries, and ideas, even possible solutions. Track your triggers and share them with someone.

Seek knowledge

What are you afraid of? Labor? Childbirth? If you are scared of labor, enroll in a labor and childbirth class or read about it online. You can watch online videos about them too. What does the body do during labor? What are the different stages of labor, and what can you do to cope with them? Understanding pregnancy and childbirth reduce your worries significantly.

In those classes, you'll learn different methods of dealing with labor pains. If you are lucky, you may even speak to other mothers who were scared about childbirth at first but eventually overcame their fears.

CHAPTER SEVEN

Strategies for Inducing Labor

A s the due date approaches, you worry about your options for labor. Maybe the due date quickly came and went, and you are googling different ways to stimulate your body and persuade the baby into action. The internet is full of information on how to coax the baby out naturally, but experts believe there are no natural, fool-proof techniques to coax your baby out except for induced labor.

However, a growing school of studies suggests that if your baby and your body cooperate, labor can be "induced" naturally using different methods. Still, the only surefire and reliable method of labor induction is medication by a healthcare provider.

What is inducing labor?

Labor is a natural process that may occur between your 37th and 42nd week of pregnancy. One of the first signs of approaching labor is; that the water breaks, contractions start, and your cervical muscles relax, becoming soft and elastic for your baby's easy and safe exit. But as we all know, babies come when they are ready, and sometimes they are just not.

Healthcare providers may decide to stimulate your labor process artificially, known as labor induction. Labor induction can be done mechanically; a doctor may break your water, open your cervix, give you medication to kick off contractions – or combine all these methods. The probability of success in induced labor is usually determined by the degree of cervical ripening – how soft and elastic it is.

Experts agree that the benefits of labor induction outweigh the risks by far.

Why is it done?

Doctors recommend labor induction for so many reasons. A doctor will suggest labor induction if there's a concern for you or your baby's health, if you had a high-risk pregnancy, if you are well past your due date or if the placenta can't support the baby enough.

The doctor must examine you and the baby before inducing labor. The examination determines if induction is safe enough for you. They will also evaluate the baby's position in the womb, the condition of your cervix, and the baby's size, weight, and gestational age.

Once all of these are determined, the healthcare provider will induce labor:

- If your pregnancy is post-term – some doctors will advise you to go for 42 weeks if you have a low-risk pregnancy; others will recommend labor induction if you are past the 41st week.

- If labor is yet to begin naturally and your water broke already, and there is evidence of membrane rupture and other signs of labor.

- If there is a significant reduction of fetal movement, changes in their heart rate, or it seems like they aren't growing well.

- Your uterus has an infection, medically known as chorioamnionitis.

- If it's a case of multiple births such as triplets, twins, or more.

- If there are signs that the baby's growth is restricted, the baby's weight is somewhere in the 10th or less of the average birth weight.

- If you have certain conditions, including issues with your kidneys, diabetes, obesity, or heart conditions.

- If you struggled with gestational diabetes during pregnancy. Gestational diabetes usually starts during pregnancy.

- If the healthcare provider determines that the placenta isn't working as expected. For example, the placenta may have peeled, either partially or entirely, from your uterine wall.

- If the amniotic fluid surrounding the baby isn't enough

- If you struggle with high blood pressure-related complications, such as having high blood pressure before pregnancy or developing high blood pressure before or after your 20th week of pregnancy.

How is it done?

Labor can be induced in multiple ways

You may be given medicines that:

- Soften the cervix and make it thinner.

- Help start uterine contractions.

- A healthcare provider may use a balloon catheter to open your cervix.

- The healthcare provider may break the amniotic fluid mechanically, especially if the cervix is slightly open already.

Sometimes, mothers are just eager to meet their babies, and they can't wait any longer. In such a case, an expectant mother may ask for induced labor for their convenience, meaning they don't need medical intervention in the first place. This is called elective labor induction. Elective labor can be helpful in other scenarios; for example, if a mother has a history of quick deliveries and doesn't live close enough to a hospital, she may opt for elective labor induction to avoid an unattended birth.

Is it painful?

Yes, the chances are that induced labor will be more painful than natural labor. That's because natural labor is intuitive, and the contractions pick up pace gradually, but the contractions in induced labor are more vigorous and quicker. You'll probably need pain relief medication.

When labor is induced, your baby's birth would require other interventions too. A pair of forceps or a ventose may be used to help deliver the baby. Doctors will monitor the birth more closely than if the birth was natural. Again, if the labor is induced, you may not move around much.

Your experience of induced labor will differ from the next mother. That's because everybody responds differently to these medications. For one mother, induced labor may take hours for one person, for another, it may take as long as two or three days. Induced labor may take longer for first-time mothers or if you are induced around the 37th week or before.

Labor induction happens in a hospital, and because it is more painful than a natural birth, various pain relief methods will be available to you. There is little to no restriction on pain relief medications you can be given when you are induced.

Induced labor is quite helpful, but it's not always an option, especially if:

- The baby is lying on their side or if they are bottom first (breech).

- You have an untreated infection such as genital herpes.

- You suffer an umbilical cord prolapse; the umbilical cord accidentally slides into the vagina before birth.

- You suffer placenta previa, which is where your placenta blocks the cervix.

- You previously had major abdominal surgery.

- You have a classical incision from a previous cesarean section.

What should you expect during labor induction?

Depending on what the healthcare provider thinks is the safest method for you and the baby, you can expect the following.

The healthcare provider will place synthetic prostaglandins inside the vagina to ripen and soften your cervix. The doctor will then monitor the baby's heart rate and contractions. Sometimes, the doctor may decide to insert a catheter with an inflated balloon inside your cervix. The balloon is filled with saline and pressed against the cervix to help ripen it.

If the doctor decides to do an amniotomy or "tear" the amniotic sac, they will use a plastic hook to create a tiny opening in your amniotic sac. You'll feel a warm fluid flowing when the sac opens and your water breaks. Amniotomy is usually done when the cervix is already thin and dilated, and the baby's head is already in the pelvic area. The doctor will monitor the baby's heartbeat during and after the amniotomy.

Alternatively, the healthcare provider may use intravenous medication. The doctor will inject you with Pitocin (synthetic oxytocin) to induce uterine contractions. Oxytocin does a better job at stepping up existent labor than inducing it. Meanwhile, the doctor will monitor your baby's heart rate continuously.

Sometimes, doctors use multiple methods to induce labor; don't be alarmed.

Are there risks associated with labor induction?

As you would expect, there are certain risks associated with labor.

Studies show that ¾ of induced first-time mothers will have successful vaginal deliveries. This means that approximately ¼ of induced mothers will end up with a c-sectional delivery. Your doctor will discuss these options with you and advise you on the best way forward.

The labor-inducing medications may not always work in your favor. The quick, unnatural, and excessive contractions may reduce the baby's heart rate and diminish their oxygen supply.

Labor induction is generally safe, but sometimes it may increase the risk of infections in you and your baby when specific methods are used.

It is infrequent, but sometimes, your uterus may rupture following the previous c-section or abdominal surgery's scar line. Such a life-threatening complication may require a c-section, and the uterus may be removed.

Labor induction may also cause excessive bleeding after delivery.

Most labor inductions lead to successful vaginal deliveries so, it will have no implications on future pregnancies and births. Suppose the induction ended with a c-section. In that case, you'll need a thorough physical examination from your doctor, followed by advice on whether or not you should attempt a vaginal delivery with your subsequent pregnancies.

Natural methods of inducing labor

If you are not a fan of induced labor, or there isn't a medical reason why you should, you can opt for natural labor induction methods. You should be extremely careful with these methods; you don't want to push a half-baked bun out of the oven, do you? Make sure your doctor or midwife has given you the green light to try the following natural methods of inducing labor.

Sex

Thinking about sex when you are heavily pregnant and almost due or overdue may sound impossible, but it's possible, and it can be helpful. This is where your partner's "services" come in handy. You may not know, but sperms have a powerful hormone called prostaglandins. This hormone can play a big part in thinning and ripening your cervix. The hormone can also stimulate cervical dilation in preparation for delivery.

Other experts disagree. Some studies report that having sex in late pregnancy could delay birth, so a sexually active woman may carry the baby longer than an inactive one.

Either way, the baby might be overdue already, so this natural method of inducing labor is worth the shot; if it doesn't work, it would still help you strengthen your muscles and relieve some tension around the pelvic area before the baby arrives.

Castor oil

Castor oil might not be delicious, but it is an efficient laxative. Women have used castor oil for thousands of years and passed down the tradition. By causing spasms, castor oil can stimulate your insides, irritate the uterus and cause contractions.

Talk to your healthcare provider before you try castor oil. It can cause stomach complications too. You are very close to delivery, and you don't want to end up in the hospital with a bad case of diarrhea.

Walking

Gravity is on your side here. Your hip movements and gravity can help pull the baby down into the pelvic area as you walk. As the baby exerts pressure on your pelvis, your cervix may start thinning and ripening for labor. Walking can also intensify labor if it's happening already.

Suppose walking doesn't help with the contraction; it is exercise and will improve your fitness level in readiness for delivery. That's a win.

Acupuncture

The thin needles inserted into your body's pressure points can spur the baby into action and the uterus into movement. Experts and expectant mothers swear that acupuncture works. Because it is a natural stress reliever, it could help.

Others argue that acupuncture alone won't convince a baby to come out if they aren't ready. So, save your money and practice a little patience. If you choose to try it anyway, consult your healthcare provider first.

Spices

Some people argue that spicy food can irritate the intestines (mildly) and cause uterine contractions. There isn't enough scientific proof to support the spicy food theory regarding labor induction. You may only end up with an upset stomach or heartburn. Always be careful.

If you don't mind spicy food and always tolerate it well, you can try it.

Acupressure

Acupressure is similar to acupuncture in many ways. Like acupuncture, acupressure has been passed down generations for thousands of years. The only difference is fingertips, instead of needles are used to exert pressure. By inserting pressure on different points in your body, acupressure could stimulate uterine contractions.

The practitioner will exert pressure inside your leg and the webbing between the index finger and thumb to induce labor naturally. Consult with your doctor before trying anything like this.

Nipple stimulation

Nipple stimulation can induce labor naturally. Try some little massage or twisting movements for a few hours every day. Nipple stimulation may cause oxytocin hormone production, which can stimulate uterine contractions.

Other healthcare providers disagree with nipple stimulation as a natural way of inducing labor, arguing that it can cause intense and painful contractions. Always consult with your doctor first.

Herbs

You can also use herbs like black cohosh, red raspberry leaf, and evening primrose oil to induce labor. There are no studies to establish their effectiveness or safety, so don't use any of them before you consult with your healthcare provider.

If you are not into anything discussed in this chapter, you can try cuddling with your partner or mindfulness and meditation practices. Cuddling and meditation calm you and stimulate oxytocin production. This could explain why labor starts late in the night for many pregnant mothers. They are relaxed, probably lying comfortably in bed, which triggers the production of the oxytocin hormone.

Try relaxing activities like meditation if you want to induce labor. Even if it doesn't induce labor, you'll significantly improve your mood and mental health.

CHAPTER EIGHT

Labor Coping methods

How do you know you're in labor? (Stages of labor)

It's difficult to tell when you're in labor. Each woman's labor is unique. It starts at different times and happens in different ways. Some symptoms may suggest that your labor will begin soon. However, labor is a process; when it starts, it could take anywhere from a few hours to days before your baby arrives.

Here are some indicators that your labor will begin soon:

Lightening

This refers to the sensation that the baby has "dropped" or moved lower in the uterus.

Its effects are:

- A tight pelvis.

- Lighter rib cage because the baby has moved further down the uterus.

- You'll breathe more easily because the baby is no longer pressing against your lungs.

- Frequent urination. This is caused by the baby pressing on your bladder.

-

Increased vaginal discharge

A mucus plug clogs the cervical opening during pregnancy, preventing microorganisms from accessing the uterus. This plug may press into your vagina during the last weeks of pregnancy (third trimester). You may notice an increase in somewhat bloody or clear vaginal discharge. This could happen a few days before or just as labor begins.

However, if your vaginal bleeding is severe, you should see your doctor immediately. Heavy vaginal bleeding may indicate a problem.

Strong, frequent contractions

If your contractions are 2 to 5 minutes apart and are getting stronger each time, preventing you from walking or even talking, you're in labor. Lower back and abdominal pain may accompany the contractions and may not be relieved by moving or changing positions.

Your water breaks

A sac of water surrounds your infant while in the womb. When this sac ruptures, the fluid leaks into the vaginal canal. You'll notice an irregular or constant trickle of fluid or a gush of fluid from your vagina. After your water has broken, the risk of infection for you and your baby increases, and it's important to get to a hospital fast.

What to expect when you're in labor

During labor, you'll notice certain changes that may cause you to panic. Understand that some of these symptoms are common and shouldn't cause alarm.

Diarrhea

As the uterine muscles relax to prepare for the baby, other muscles in your body, including the rectal muscles, also relax. Relaxation of the anal sphincter muscles causes diarrhea.

Though annoying, pre-labor diarrhea is entirely normal and is a good sign. Just remember to stay hydrated.

Gaining weight stops

During labor, you may lose a couple of pounds. Don't be alarmed. It is normal because of the frequent water breaks.

Nesting instinct and fatigue

Getting a decent night's sleep in the last days or weeks of pregnancy can be difficult. Your belly is huge, and you are working with a constricted bladder, cramped pelvic muscles and organs. Pile up your pillows and take naps whenever you can.

You may get a sudden urge to clean everything in sight as you prepare for your baby. This is called nesting instinct and is normal.

Lax joints

Before going into labor, your body releases relaxin hormones. This hormone calms your body down, leading to muscle relaxation in preparation for delivery. You'll notice that your joints are less tense and painful. It's nature's way of allowing your little angel to enter the world through your pelvis.

Steps to cope with labor

Pain during labor is normal. But what can you do when the agony is real and the pain unbearable?

There are three stages of labor based on the physiological processes happening in the cervix: The early, active transitional labor, childbirth, and delivery of the placenta.

Understanding how to cope with labor pain during these three stages is crucial.

Stage 1: The early, active transitional labor

What happens? The cervix opens and shortens, causing recurrent contractions at this stage. The process lasts for hours or even days.

How to cope:

- Take a warm shower

- Go for a walk

- Listen to soothing music

- Change positions

- Write a letter to your baby

- Practice breathing techniques

Stage 2: Childbirth

This is the delivery or "pushing" stage.

How long does it last? Pushing your baby might take a few minutes to several hours. Studies show that many first time mothers and those who've had epidurals have longer labor.

How to cope:

- Request for a mirror so that you can see your baby as he comes out

- Relax your pelvis

- Take subsequent breaths when pushing

- Use a birthing ball

- Kneel, stand, or squat to ease up things

Stage 3: Delivery of the placenta
The tough part is over; this is the final and easiest part.

What happens? Mild contractions will occur, and the midwife will request you to push out the placenta.

How to cope:

Enjoy every second with your baby. It's the moment you've been waiting for!

What you might be feeling

You will experience many emotions after childbirth; this is normal.

Here are some common feelings you may have soon after giving birth:

Pain

After-delivery uterine contractions generate cramp-like, afterbirth symptoms. The uterus begins to contract shortly after childbirth. These contractions may last for six weeks before the uterus returns to its former size and placement.

Oxytocin, the hormone responsible for involution, is produced in greater quantities immediately after delivery when the agony is at its peak. This hormone is also released during breastfeeding.

As a result, postpartum pain is likely to occur while nursing.

Fatigue

Delivery is hard work, so fatigue is expected. Postpartum fatigue may affect your ability to take care of the baby or even yourself. It can also make it difficult to get enough sleep, exacerbating the problem.

Relief

You'll be relieved to know that the most difficult part is now behind you and everything went smoothly.

Joy

There's nothing like the joy of announcing your baby's arrival to your loved ones and the world. It's also exciting to watch your family members get ecstatic when they eventually meet the baby.

Fear

You may be scared that you or other people will accidentally hurt the baby. You'll be on high alert and may even struggle with intrusive thoughts about your baby falling or choking. This fear will go away with time; just try to relax.

How can your partner help?

There are numerous practical things that your birth partner (the baby's father, a close friend, or family) can do to assist you.

Your birth partner's most vital role is to be physically and emotionally present with you. Their emotional presence allows you to take a mental vacation from caring for your precious child. Their physical presence allows you to take care of yourself. Your basic human needs must be satisfied, and you must replenish your energy.

Your birth partner can help you in the following ways:

Monitoring your mood

Up to 80% of new mothers experience postpartum depression, and these troubling feelings usually subside after two weeks. If you're still feeling overwhelmed several weeks after the baby arrives, your spouse can encourage you to speak with your practitioner. Postpartum depression is a serious problem that requires urgent medical intervention.

Help with babysitting

Since you're recovering after the delivery, your partner can visit the crib and allow you to nap. Taking turns to babysit is a crucial bonding time for you all.

Cook

After delivery, roles change, and you won't be making frequent trips to the kitchen as before. Your partner can help by preparing a balanced diet for you. This is the time to regain strength by sticking to a healthy diet.

Different pain medicines to consider

Your body will need time to recuperate after giving birth. After delivery, the most frequent symptom is pain, which can last anywhere from a few days to a few weeks. Self-help remedies, over-the-counter drugs, and prescription medicine are some options for pain management.

Common pain management drugs include;

Nitrous oxide

Nitrous oxide is an odorless, tasteless gas given through a hand-held face mask. It takes effect within sixty seconds.

Paracetamol

This drug is used for mild-to-moderate pain. It has few side effects and is suitable for mothers with stomach ulcers.

Anti-inflammatory drugs

These include ibuprofen, aspirin, meloxicam, and mefenamic acid. After delivery, the tissues around the uterus and vagina become inflamed because of excessive stretching. Anti-inflammatories fight inflammation and reduce swelling and pain.

You shouldn't take these drugs if you have ulcers because they can erode stomach walls. You can opt for celecoxib or etoricoxib, which fight inflammation and don't cause peptic ulcers.

Opioids

These are stronger painkillers. Some examples are pethidine, morphine, and tramadol. They are more effective when combined with paracetamol and an anti-inflammatory drug. Because of the risk of addiction, you should take opioids in low doses and for a very short time, preferably not more than one week.

The advantages and disadvantages of pain medication

Drugs have pros and cons, and pain medications are not an exception. As a mother, it is advisable to seek your doctor's opinion before taking any medication. Some medications pass through breast milk and may be harmful to your baby.

The following are common pain medications, advantages, and disadvantages.

Delivery without pain medication

Pain medications are beneficial because they speed up delivery, but they may have side effects. Most women choose natural birth because it gives them more control over the birthing process, including pain management. They believe pain medication may cloud their memory when they prefer to remember the event vividly and bond with their child during delivery.

Women with low-risk pregnancies can deliver without pain medication.

A high-risk pregnancy needs medical intervention and is necessary especially:

- If you're older than 35 years

- You're an alcoholic

- You have a previous history of cesarean section

- You have a medical history of diabetes or hypertension

- You're carrying twins or triplets

- You have a history of complications during delivery

- The baby has macrocephaly (larger than normal head)

- The baby is lying in a breech or transverse position

- If a mother has a sexually transmitted infection, like syphilis

Delivery without pain medication takes longer and is more painful. If you choose natural birth, you'll need to practice the following pain relief methods:

- Breathing techniques

- Using a birthing ball

- Choose a position you find most comfortable

- Emotional support

- Massage

- An ice pack or hot packs

Remember that having a natural childbirth without medication is empowering. Once you get through it, you can get through anything in life.

Natural birth vs C-section

Between these two delivery methods, none is better than the other. The main difference is that one is done by choice, while the other may be medically necessary. Both have pros and cons, but ultimately only you as a mother can choose which delivery method works best for you.

Natural birth

Recommended if you have a low-risk pregnancy.

Advantages

- Fast recovery

- Fewer risks of infection

- No scarring

- Lesser medications

- Babies need shorter monitoring

- Quicker bonding between the mother and her baby

- Shorter hospital stay

Risks

- More painful

- Hemorrhoids

- Weakening of pelvic muscles

- Skin tearing

- Painful bowel movements

Cesarean/ C-section

Recommended if you have a high-risk pregnancy.

Advantages

- Less pain

- Saves lives

- Lower injury risks to the baby

- Fewer sexual problems

Risks

- Longer hospital stay

- Longer recovery period

- Higher death rates

- Adhesions

- Higher risks of infection

- Postpartum depression

- Surgical accidents

- Anesthetic complications

- Increased risk of bleeding

Chapter Nine

Recovering from Delivery

What to expect in the birth room?

If you have a normal delivery, your baby will be placed on your chest right away for skin-to-skin contact. The benefits of skin-to-skin contact include:

- It relaxes both you and your child

- It regulates your baby's heart rate

- It regulates your baby's temperature

- Skin-to-skin contact allows your friendly bacteria to colonize the baby's skin, protecting your baby against infection.

- Skin-to-skin contact enhances the release of hormones that stimulate breastfeeding.

Suppose you've experienced complications during normal delivery or had a c-section. In that case, the midwife will use a radiant warmer to keep your baby warm while your doctor examines your baby's condition and performs tests. You shouldn't be worried, though — you'll get your skin-to-skin bonding eventually.

Your doctor will perform the Apgar test on your newborn shortly after birth to assess the general status and see whether there are any acute health problems. This test will be conducted within the first minute of birth and repeated after 5 minutes. The one-minute test checks if the baby tolerated the birthing process well. The five-minute test checks how the baby is doing outside the womb.

The overall goal of the test is to inspect whether or not your baby requires any additional medical attention after birth. It is not a diagnosis or a prognosis for your baby's long-term health. It's simply a way for the doctor to evaluate if and what immediate medical attention is required.

Shortly after birth, babies typically open their eyes for the first time, and they are highly alert during the first hour. The nurses in the delivery room will apply an antibiotic ointment to your baby's eyes, which can cause short-term blurriness, but you can ask them to wait a few minutes while you bond.

The first hour after delivery is the opportune time to breastfeed your baby. Not only is it an excellent way to bond, but your baby also benefits from colostrum. Colostrum is the initial, highly nutritious fluid before breast milk.

The first 24 hours

Soon after delivery, there are some common postpartum symptoms women experience in the first 24 hours:

Breast engorgement

Breast engorgement is when the breasts swell and become painful and tender. It occurs a few hours after childbirth and is caused by increased blood flow and milk production in your breasts.

Breast engorgement should subside after two to three days if you breastfeed continuously.

How to manage:

- Before nursing, use warm compresses to soften the areola and cold compresses after that.

- Breastfeed every three hours to relieve pressure from your breasts.

- Express a little milk with your hand to ease some pressure. But don't express too much because it will make things worse.

- Put on a well-fitting bra.

- Consider pain medications prescribed by your doctor if the pain is unbearable.

Constipation

Causes of postpartum constipation include:

- Injury to the pelvic floor and rectal muscles because of excessive stretching during delivery.

- Dehydration, especially if you did not take enough water or vomited a lot during labor.

- The release of hormones during delivery may slow down bowel function.

- Perineal pain following episiotomy (vaginal surgical cut to aid delivery) may cause you to retain stool because of the fear of tearing stitches.

- Postpartum hemorrhoids (swollen veins around the anus) cause intense pain when passing stool, so you may try to hold it in to avoid the pain.

- Excessive use of opioids for pain management during delivery causes constipation.

To manage postpartum constipation, drink plenty of water, take pain medication, don't retain stool, eat foods high in fiber, and go for walks.

Hot and cold flashes

Postpartum flashes may occur a few hours after giving birth. You may feel hot on your chest, shoulders, face, and neck. This is often accompanied by redness and excessive sweating in the affected areas. Chills may accompany the overwhelming heat, making you feel both cold and hot.

A decrease in estrogen levels affects the temperature-regulating center in your brain, causing postpartum flashes. It may last for about six weeks and is accompanied by fatigue and insomnia.

How to manage:

- Use a fan or air conditioner to keep cool, but do not expose the baby to the cold.

- Drink plenty of water to stay hydrated.

- Avoid spicy foods, alcohol, and hot foods.

- Manage stress using relaxation techniques, like, deep breathing exercises and meditation.

Hemorrhoids

These are swollen veins around the anus caused by too much pressure on the perineum before and after delivery. The perineum is the space between the anus and vulva. Its functions are to protect, contain, and support the abdominal and pelvic organs, including the uterus. Hemorrhoids can also be caused by straining when passing stool, chronic diarrhea, and obesity.

How to manage:

- Take pain relief medication prescribed by your doctor.

- Use fiber supplements or eat foods high in fiber.

- Wash your anus using plain warm water; don't use soap.

- After passing the stool, don't use dry tissue paper; you can use soft padding or cotton wool soaked in water.

Baby blues

The baby blues, also known as postpartum blues, are emotions of sadness that most women experience after giving birth. It usually kicks in hours after delivery and can stay for a couple of weeks. The good news is that baby blues often go away without the need for any particular intervention or medicine.

It is accompanied by anxiety, irritability, loss of appetite, and insomnia. The causes of baby blues are:

- Decrease in estrogen levels after giving birth.

- A tough delivery.

- Feelings of guilt and shock when you see the baby. You might be experiencing conflicting feelings about your new responsibility as a parent.

Baby blues differs from postpartum depression in that the latter lasts more than two weeks.

How to manage: Socializing is the best and most effective way to get rid of baby blues. Engage your partner, friends, or family and pour your heart out.

The healing process between vaginal delivery and C-section

Every birth is unique, just like every pregnancy. Some women take pain relievers, while others don't. Some labor for a few hours, while others take longer. Some women give birth vaginally, while others have their babies via C-section.

The recovery period for vaginal delivery and c-section is not the same for every woman and depends on many factors.

C-section recovery

C-section necessitates a lot of medication during recovery. Following a C-section, lots of activities are restricted. For around six weeks after this surgery, a woman should not lift anything heavier than her infant. She should be assisted in the house, including taking care of her other children if any. She should not drive for at least two weeks or while under narcotics.

Women who went through tough labor before a C-section usually take the longest to recuperate. They need to recover from the surgery and labor as well.

C-sections don't affect weight after delivery; nevertheless, a prolonged period of being less active makes weight loss more difficult.

Vaginal birth recovery

Recovery time is significantly reduced because surgery is not required. Pain and discomfort normally persist for a few weeks, although you can manage with over-the-counter pain relievers. Typically, your doctor will advise you to refrain from intense exercise for six weeks to aid in the healing of your pelvic floor muscles.

While there are exceptions, vaginal birth is generally easier on the body than a c-section, with a quicker recovery time and a shorter hospital stay of less than two days compared to a c-section, whose hospital stay is around (2-4 days).

What is normal

Bleeding

After giving birth, you will notice vaginal discharge and bleeding. It's called lochia and is completely normal. When you bring your kid home, you could bleed a little more. If it occurs, take some time to rest.

It's also common to experience a gush of blood when standing. This is due to the shape of your vaginal canal. While sitting or lying down, blood gathers in a cup-like area and comes out when you stand.

Vaginal soreness

You may experience vaginal and perineal soreness for a few weeks if you had a vaginal delivery after an episiotomy. If there was severe tearing, recovery time could be longer. Place soft cushions between your thighs and take over-the-counter pain medicine to address this symptom.

Incontinence

Some urine leakage may occur after giving birth due to pelvic floor weakness throughout pregnancy, labor, and vaginal delivery. This usually improves after a few weeks, but it could last longer.

Hemorrhoids

Hemorrhoids (swollen veins around the anus) are common, especially if you're obese. They cause painful bowel movements but resolve in a couple of weeks.

Abdominal pain and cramps

You may experience lower abdominal pain as your uterus returns to its usual size. These stomach cramps are most common in the days following birth but subside as you heal.

When to call the doctor/warning signs

Postpartum hemorrhage

Postpartum hemorrhage is the term for heavy bleeding after delivery, and it affects up to 5% of women in the first 24 hours post-delivery. It is a dangerous condition because it can result in a significant reduction in blood pressure.

When your blood pressure drops too low, the organs of your body will not receive enough blood. This is called shock, and it's a medical emergency because it can be fatal.

You should call your doctor if the bleeding is accompanied by blurred vision, dizziness, blood clots, weakness, and chills.

Postpartum urinary incontinence

Urinary incontinence following delivery is normal. After delivery, weak pelvic floor muscles can cause loss of bladder control.

Urinary incontinence may be prolonged if some nerves were injured following an episiotomy. This will require urgent intervention by a medical specialist.

Breast discomfort and pain

Mild breast discomfort for a few days due to engorgement is normal. However, if the pain lasts more than a week and is accompanied by fever, flu-like symptoms, breast swelling, and redness, contact your doctor immediately; it could be mastitis.

Swelling of the legs and feet

Postpartum edema usually goes away within a week as your body gets rid of pregnancy fluid. However, if the swelling persists, it could be deep venous thrombosis (DVT), a condition where blood clots in veins, especially veins in the legs.

DVT is common soon after delivery and is usually accompanied by pain, swelling, and tenderness. The clot can travel to the lungs, causing a pulmonary embolism, which is fatal.

Postpartum depression

Baby blues/postpartum blues is normal in 80% of women after giving birth. Baby blues usually fade as hormone levels normalize; if they persist for more than a few weeks or are accompanied by other symptoms (such as insomnia or reduced appetite), you may be suffering from postpartum depression.

Contact your doctor if you have trouble sleeping at night, crying frequently, severe mood swings, trouble bonding with the baby, and confusion.

How to take care of myself

The postpartum phase begins after your baby is delivered and ends when your body is practically back to its pre-pregnancy form. This stage usually lasts six to eight weeks.

Here are some post-delivery healing techniques to help you get back on your feet after your baby is born.

Rest

In the first few weeks, you should be liberated of all responsibilities except feeding your baby, taking care of yourself, and sleeping. Getting plenty of rest aids in speedy recovery.

Nutrition

When you're hungry and don't have time to cook, you may grab whatever is convenient, but this is wrong. After delivery, eating a well-balanced meal is essential for speedy healing and vigor. You'll need that extra energy even more if you're breastfeeding! Making milk burns more calories than giving birth.

Drink plenty of water

Water keeps your body functioning properly, so drink enough of it, especially if you're breastfeeding. Constipation will be relieved, and you'll stay hydrated. If you have difficulties drinking enough water, get a water bottle that keeps track of your intake. You can also download a water-tracking app.

Express yourself

Hormonal changes post-delivery can be such a rollercoaster. Don't be concerned if you're frequently stressed or depressed. It will pass in a few weeks, so express yourself to your partner or parents for support.

Contact your doctor

Call your doctor if you experience excruciating pain or anything abnormal.

Conclusion

For a baby to be born healthy, the mother must be healthy, physically and mentally. If a mother is not happy and healthy, a baby may be affected even before birth. For this reason, we can conclude that there is nothing more critical than prenatal and postnatal health for every pregnant mother. Without awareness and the proper physical and maternal mental health, a mother would be incapable of loving, caring, delivering, and raising a healthy child.

You play an important role in your unborn baby's health and overall quality of life. Don't miss out on any prenatal appointments because you and your baby's health should be a priority during pregnancy. Doctors can monitor you and the baby and deal with existing or new health complications on time if you prioritize a healthy pregnancy.

Your body will change throughout the trimesters. Some changes might be expected, others, not so much. While some symptoms cut across, others may be unique because every woman's pregnancy experiences are different.

Chapter 1 highlights what you should expect in terms of how your body reacts during each stage of pregnancy. Pregnancy will affect your emotions too. You'll frequently find yourself on extreme ends of the emotional scale – happiness and sadness. That's completely normal.

Multiple studies report that up to 15% of women struggle with the realities of pregnancy and may experience anxiety, depression, or both. You must create a strong-knit support system now. 95% of expectant mothers have access to the internet and use it to find information relating to childbirth and pregnancy, according to one Swedish study.

64% of those women struggle with needless anxiety after "consulting" Dr. Google. The same study reports a direct relationship between online searches and contacting doctors or midwives by pregnant mothers. The more online searches you do, the more likely you will call a healthcare provider with panic-stricken questions relating to pregnancy and birth.

It's necessary for you as a mother to filter what you consume. Look for reliable sources of information that you can trust; not every blog you find online is authentic or dependable.

It's important to understand that most women go through pregnancy and labor without issues. Most of them will have normal vaginal deliveries and will heal quickly. If you are healthy and have a non-complicated pregnancy, there's no need to worry.

However, make sure you are well prepared for your baby's arrival. Chapter 3 discusses the need to find a reliable healthcare provider and the steps you can take to find one. You must prepare for the baby's arrival and get everything ready; the hospital bag, birth plan, plan for expected and unexpected expenses, insurance coverage, and how your older kids, if you have any, will be taken care of when you deliver.

Pregnancy will take a toll on you; it's best to turn to a healthy, nutritious diet, so you have enough strength for delivery and give birth to a healthy baby with no health complications.

Analyze your diet at this time and eat things that favor your baby's health. Fitness and exercise should be part of your healthy pregnancy lifestyle too. Find manageable exercises that you can do, even in the comfort of your home. You can find simple, pregnancy-related fitness videos online.

As discussed in Chapter 6, mindfulness and meditation give pregnant women relief from anxiety and pregnancy-related stresses. Be present at this moment because you don't get to live a pregnancy twice, at least not with this baby.

Slow down when you need to and meditate to calm yourself down where necessary. Take control of your thoughts; it's the only way to stay sane during your 40-week pregnancy journey.

A follow-up study of the Swedish study mentioned above reported that 32% of women who had vaginal births and 62% of those who had assisted births admitted that they weren't well informed about labor and childbirth. Empower yourself with knowledge about labor and how to cope with it, as discussed in Chapters 7 and 8. With access to factual, truthful, and reliable information, you'll be better placed to make informed choices about medicalization during labor and childbirth.

You have a responsibility to your body, your health, and your baby's health. You must be adequately informed and well advised about pregnancy and everything relating to it. I hope this book has helped provide you with information about pregnancy, nutrition, exercise, labor, delivery, recovery, and everything in between. Use everything you have learned and ask for professional advice when unsure.

1.   Victoria State Government. (2012, December 28). *Pregnancy Week by Week.* Better Health Channel. Retrieved May 16, 2022, from

2.   Geddes, J. K. G. (2021, February 22). *Your Guide to Prenatal Appointments.* Everyday Health. Retrieved May 16, 2022, from https://www.whattoexpect.com/pregnancy/pregnancy-health/prenatal-appointments/

3.   Grow by WebMD. (n.d.). *Pregnancy's Emotional Roller Coaster.* WebMD. Retrieved May 16, 2022, from https://www.webmd.com/baby/features/pregnancy-emotional-roller-coaster

4.   *Month by Month.* (n.d.). Planned Parenthood. Retrieved May 16, 2022, from https://www.plannedparenthood.org/learn/pregnancy/pregnancy-month-by-month

5.   North Texas Medical Center. (2020, February 6). *5 TIPS TO MENTALLY & PHYSICALLY PREPARE FOR CHILDBIRTH.* Retrieved May 16, 2022, from https://ntmconline.net/how-to-prepare-for-delivering-a-baby/

6.   Riley, L. R. (2009, November 2). *10 Tips to Ease Your Fear of Childbirth.* Parents. Retrieved May 16, 2022, from

https://www.parents.com/pregnancy/my-life/emotions/conquering-fears-of-childbirth/

7. Kernodle Clinic. (n.d.). *Preparing for Baby: 10 Things to Do Before You Give Birth*. Kernodle.Com. Retrieved May 16, 2022, from https://www.kernodle.com/obgyn_blog/preparing-for-baby/

8. Booth, S. B. (n.d.). *How to Prepare for a Baby: What I Wish I Knew*. WebMD. Retrieved May 16, 2022, from https://www.webmd.com/parenting/baby/features/prepare-for-baby

9. 9 Super Easy Mindfulness Exercises For A Calmer and More Enjoyable Pregnancy. (n.d.). Baby Doppler Blog. Retrieved May 16, 2022, from https://www.babydoppler.com/blog/9-super-easy-mindfulness-exercises-for-a-calmer-and-more-enjoyable-pregnancy/

10. Collier 2021, S. C. (2021, June 25). *How can you manage anxiety during pregnancy?* Harvard Health Publishing. Retrieved May 16, 2022, from https://www.health.harvard.edu/blog/how-can-you-manage-anxiety-during-pregnancy-202106252512

11. Bellefonds, C. B. (2022, January 25). *Natural Ways to Induce Labor*. Everyday Health. Retrieved May 16, 2022, from

https://www.whattoexpect.com/pregnancy/photo-gallery/natural-ways-to-induce-labor.aspx

12.   Mayo Clinic Staff. (2020, May 13). *Labor Induction*. Mayo Clinic. Retrieved May 16, 2022, from https://www.mayoclinic.org/tests-procedures/labor-induction/about/pac-20385141

13.   Health Wise Staff. (2022, February 23). *Labor Induction and Augmentation*. Health Wise. Retrieved May 16, 2022, from https://www.peacehealth.org/medical-topics/id/hw194662

14.   Rauh, S. R. (2020, August 6). *Natural Ways to Induce Labor*. WebMD. Retrieved May 16, 2022, from https://www.webmd.com/baby/inducing-labor-naturally-can-it-be-done

15.   10 Surprising Things to Expect After Giving Birth. (2017, July 25). Mombrite. Retrieved May 11, 2022, from https://www.mombrite.com/things-to-expect-after-giving-birth/

16.   1900 Ways to Support During Labor | A Partner's Treasure Trove of Tips and Tricks. (2018, March 20). Baby Nest Birth Services; babynestbirth.com. Retrieved May 11, 2022 from https://babynestbirth.com/2018/03/20/100-ways-a-partner-can-support-during-labor/

17.   236 Ways to Support Your Partner Before, During, and After Birth. (2020, May 18). Pregnant Chicken. Retrieved May 11, 2022, from https://pregnantchicken.com/supporting-partner-birth/

18.   Benefits and Side Effects of IV Medications Used for Pain in Labor. (2021, June 14). Verywell Family. Retrieved   May   11,   2021   from https://www.verywellfamily.com/iv-medications-for-pain-in-labor-2759370

19.   Brewster, A. (2020, January 10). How to support your wife or partner after birth. Today's Parents. Retrieved   May   11,   2022,   from https://www.todaysparent.com/baby/postpartum-care/how-to-support-your-wife-after-birth/

20.   Coping Skills for Labor without Medication. (2018, September 4). Cleveland Clinic. Retrieved May 11, 2022,   from https://my.clevelandclinic.org/health/articles/15586-labor-without-medication-coping-skills

21.   C-Section Versus Vaginal Birth - 1707 Words | Studymode. (2013, May 24). Studymode. Retrieved May 11, 2022, from

22.   C-Section Vs Natural Birth: Which is Better? - BabyMomsy. (2020, August 19). BabyMomsy. Retrieved

May 11, 2022, from https://www.babymomsy.com/labor/c-section-vs-natural-birth/

23.   c-section vs natural birth - Bing video. (n.d.). C-Section vs Natural Birth - Bing Video; www.bing.com. Retrieved May 11, 2022, from https://www.bing.com/videos/search?q=c-section+vs+natural+birth&qpvt=c-section+vs+natural+birth&FORM=VDRE

24.   Do you feel immediately back to normal after giving birth? (2021, July 27). What to Expect. Retrieved May 11, 2022, from https://community.whattoexpect.com/forums/july-2021-babies/topic/do-you-feel-immediately-back-to-normal-after-giving-birth-117280421.html

25.   How Dads Can Help New Mothers After Baby's Birth | BellyBelly. (2006, March 20). BellyBelly. Retrieved May, 11, 2022, from https://www.bellybelly.com.au/men/how-you-can-help-mum-after-your-babys-birth/

26.   How Do I Know I Am In Labor? (2020, January 14). Familydoctor. Retrieved May 11, 2022, from

27.   How to tell if you're in labor. (2021, June 12). Allina Health. Retrieved May 11, 2022, from https://www.allinahealth.org/health-conditions-and-trea

tments/health-library/patient-education/beginnings/giving-birth/how-to-tell-if-you-are-in-labor

28.   How Will You Handle Your Labor Pain? (2020, December 4). WebMD. Retrieved May 11, 200, from.

29.   How You Can Help | Pregnancy, Birth and Beyond | Allina Health. (2021, June 12). How You Can Help | Pregnancy, Birth and Beyond | Allina Health; www.allinahealth.org. Retrieved May 11, 2022, from

30.   Labor and delivery: Pain medications. (2020, May 6). Mayo Clinic. Retrieved May 11, 2022, from https://www.mayoclinic.org/healthy-lifestyle/labor-and-delivery/in-depth/labor-and-delivery/art-20049326

31.   Mum's first 24 hours after birth | Pregnancy Birth and Baby. (n.d.). Mum's First 24 Hours after Birth | Pregnancy   Birth   and   Baby; www.pregnancybirthbaby.org.au. Retrieved May 11, 2022,   from https://www.pregnancybirthbaby.org.au/mums-first-24-hours-after-birth

32.   RunJumpScrap. (2020, July 22). Help After Birth - What can Partners Do To Help in The Newborn Days? Run Jump Scrap. Retrieved May 11, 2022, from https://runjumpscrap.com/2020/07/what-can-partners-do-to-help-after-birth/

33.   Signs of Labor: 11 Early Signs & Symptoms. (2021, August 6). What to Expect. Retrieved May 11, 2022, from https://www.whattoexpect.com/pregnancy/labor-signs

34.   Signs of labor: Know what to expect. (2021, December 16). Mayo Clinic. Retrieved May 11, 2002, f   r   o   m https://www.mayoclinic.org/healthy-lifestyle/labor-and-delivery/in-depth/signs-of-labor/art-20046184

35.   Signs of Labor: Signs & Symptoms Labor Is Near. (2022, April 15). Pampers. Retrieved May 11, 2022, from https://www.pampers.com/en-us/pregnancy/giving-birth/article/signs-symptoms-of-labor

36.   Signs You're Going Into Labor. (2022, January 4). Motherhood Incoming. Retrieved May 11, 2022, from https://www.motherhoodincoming.com/post/signs-youre-going-into-labor

37.   The Stages of Labor and Ways to Cope. (2020, October 13). Texas Health Resources. Retrieved May 11, 2022,   from https://areyouawellbeing.texashealth.org/the-stages-of-labor-and-ways-to-cope/

38.   Top 15 Ways to Reduce Labor Pain and Cope with Contractions. (2020, May 16). MIDWIFICAL. Retrieved   May   11,   2022,   from

https://midwifical.com/top-15-ways-to-reduce-labor-pain-cope-with-contractions/

39. Ways to Cope with Labor Pain. (2021, June 14). Verywell Family. Retrieved May 11, 2022, from https://www.verywellfamily.com/ways-to-cope-with-labor-2753069

40. What are the options for pain relief during labor and delivery? | NICHD - Eunice Kennedy Shriver National Institute of Child Health and Human Development. 2017, September. Retrieved May 11, 2022, from https://www.nichd.nih.gov/health/topics/labor-delivery/topicinfo/pain-relief

41. Unmedicated vs Medicated Birth. (2020, April 16). Healthline. Retrieved May 11, 2022, from https://www.healthline.com/health/pregnancy/pain-relief-in-labor

42. *5 Common Postpartum Symptoms to NEVER Ignore* (2017, August 25). Doulas of Bellingham. Retrieved May 13, 2022, from https://www.doulasofbellingham.com/5-common-postpartum-symptoms-never-ignore/

43. *5 Self-Care Tips For After Giving Birth* (2017, October 30). Tri-City Medical Center. Retrieved May 13, 2022, from

https://www.tricitymed.org/2017/10/5-self-care-tips-giv
ing-birth/

44. *6 Postpartum Symptoms You Shouldn't Neglect.*
(2022, February 17). Flo.Health. Retrieved May 13, 2022,
from
https://flo.health/being-a-mom/recovering-from-birth/p
ostpartum-problems/postpartum-symptoms

45. *8 postpartum symptoms and conditions to watch for
after delivery.* (2019, November 18). Today's Parent.
Retrieved   May   13,   2022,   from
https://www.todaysparent.com/baby/postpartum-care/p
ostpartum-symptoms-after-delivery/

46. *Don't Ignore These Postpartum Symptoms. (n.d.)*
North Pointe OB/GYN: Gynecologists. Retrieved May
13,   2022,   from
https://www.npobgyn.com/blog/dont-ignore-these-post
partum-symptoms

47. *How to Recover From a C-section.* (2020, September
21). WebMD. Retrieved May 13, 2022, from

48. *Mum's first 24 hours after birth | Pregnancy, Birth
and Baby.* (n.d.). Mum's First 24 Hours after Birth |
Pregnancy, Birth and Baby. Retrieved May 13, 2022, from

49. *Postpartum care: After a vaginal delivery.* (2022,
March 25). Mayo Clinic. Retrieved May 13, 2022, from

https://www.mayoclinic.org/healthy-lifestyle/labor-and-delivery/in-depth/postpartum-care/art-20047233

50. *Postpartum Care: Caring for Your Health After Childbirth* (n.d). Cleveland Clinic. Retrieved May 13, 2022, from https://my.clevelandclinic.org/health/articles/9679-postpartum-care

51. *Postpartum Care: Tips for the Recovery Process*. (2016, December 20). Healthline. Retrieved May 13, 2022, from https://www.healthline.com/health/postpartum-care

52. *Postnatal symptoms you should never ignore* - (2021, march). BabyCentre UK. Retrieved May 13, 2022, from https://www.babycentre.co.uk/a1011242/postnatal-symptoms-you-should-never-ignore

53. *Recovering From Delivery - Postpartum Recovery* (2017, January 26). Familydoctor.Org. Retrieved May 13, 2022, from https://familydoctor.org/recovering-from-delivery/

54. *The 24 Hours After Giving Birth* (2005, October 3). Parents. Retrieved May 13, 2022, from https://www.parents.com/pregnancy/my-body/postpartum/the-24-hours-after-giving-birth/

55. The New Mother: Taking Care of Yourself After Birth (n.d). Stanfordchildren. Retrieved May 13, 2022,

f   r   o   m
https://www.stanfordchildrens.org/en/topic/default?id=
the-new-mother-taking-care-of-yourself-after-birth-90-P
02693

56. *Top tips: taking care of yourself after having a baby.*
(2021, January 20). NCT (National Childbirth Trust).
Retrieved May 13, 2022, from www.nct.org.uk.
https://www.nct.org.uk/life-parent/self-care-and-well-be
ing/top-tips-taking-care-yourself-after-having-baby

57. *Vaginal birth vs. C-Section: Pros & cons* (2021, May
20). Livescience. Retrieved May, 13, 2022, from
https://www.livescience.com/45681-vaginal-birth-vs-c-se
ction.html

58. *Vaginal Birth After Cesarean Delivery (2021, August 2021).* NCBI
Bookshelf. Retrieved May 13, 2022, from
https://www.ncbi.nlm.nih.gov/books/NBK507844/

50. *Warning signs of postpartum complications. (2021, March 29).* BabyCenter. Retrieved May 13, 2022, from
https://www.babycenter.com/baby/postpartum-health/p
ostpartum-warning-signs_12257

60. *What Postpartum Symptoms Can I Expect After Giving Birth?* (2021, September 15). What to expect.
Retrieved   May13,   2022,   from

https://www.whattoexpect.com/first-year/postpartum-symptoms.aspx

61. *What to expect after a C-section?* (2022, April 6). Mayo Clinic. Retrieved May 13, 2022, from https://www.mayoclinic.org/healthy-lifestyle/labor-and-delivery/in-depth/c-section-recovery/art-20047310

62. *What to expect in the first 24 hours after having a baby.* (n.d.). Emma's Diary. Retrieved May 13, 2022, from https://www.emmasdiary.co.uk/baby/new-born-care/what-to-expect-in-the-first-24-hours-after-having-a-baby

63. *Your baby's first 24 hours: What to expect after birth.* (2020, November 10). GoodtoKnow. Retrieved May 13, 2022, from https://www.goodto.com/family/babies/babys-first-24-hours-72183

64. *Your first 24 hours after having a baby | Queensland Health.* (2019, May 29). Retrieved May 13, 2022, from https://www.health.qld.gov.au/news-events/news/your-first-24-hours-after-having-a-baby-postpartum-postnatal

65. *541 Foods and Beverages to Avoid During Pregnancy.* (n.d.). Healthline. Retrieved May 12, 2022, from https://www.healthline.com/nutrition/11-foods-to-avoid-during-pregnancy

66. Cheatham, C. L. (2020, June 19). *Nutritional Factors in Fetal and Infant Brain Development - FullText - Annals of Nutrition and Metabolism 2019, Vol. 75, Suppl. 1 - Karger Publishers*. Nutritional Factors in Fetal and Infant Brain Development - FullText - Annals of Nutrition and Metabolism 2019, Vol. 75, Suppl. 1 - Karger Publishers; www.karger.com. https://www.karger.com/Article/FullText/508052

67. *Current Concepts of Maternal Nutrition - PMC*. (2016, July 1). PubMed Central (PMC); Retrieved May 12, 2022, from. https://www.ncbi.nlm.nih.gov/pmc/articles/PMC49490 06/

68. *Do you know which foods to avoid when you're pregnant?* (2022, January 22). Mayo Clinic. Retrieved May 12, 2022, from https://www.mayoclinic.org/healthy-lifestyle/pregnancy-week-by-week/in-depth/pregnancy-nutrition/art-200438 44

69. *Food Safety for Pregnant Women*. (2021, October 28). U.S. Food and Drug Administration. Retrieved May 12, 2022, from https://www.fda.gov/food/people-risk-foodborne-illness /food-safety-pregnant-women-and-their-unborn-babies

70. *Foods to avoid in pregnancy*. (n.d.). Nhs.Uk. Retrieved May 12, 2022, from https://www.nhs.uk/pregnancy/keeping-well/foods-to-avoid/

71. *Foods to avoid when pregnant*. (n.d.). Pregnancy Birth and Baby. Retrieved May 12, 2022, from https://www.pregnancybirthbaby.org.au/foods-to-avoid-when-pregnant

72. *Healthy Eating Guidelines for Food Safety During Pregnancy*. (n.d.). HealthLink BC. Retrieved May 12, 2022, from https://www.healthlinkbc.ca/pregnancy-parenting/pregnancy/healthy-eating-and-physical-activity/healthy-eating-guidelines-food

73. *How Nutrition and Weight Gain Affect Your Pregnancy and Baby*. (2021, June 14). Verywell Family. Retrieved May 12, 2022, from https://www.verywellfamily.com/nutrition-during-pregnancy-4172730

74. *Impact of Maternal Nutrition on Fetal Development*. (n.d.). Mednet. Retrieved May 12, 2022, from https://www.mednet.ca/en/report/impact-of-maternal-nutrition-on-fetal-developmen.html

75. *Malnutrition in Pregnancy: Causes, Health Risks & Prevention.* (2018, July 12). FirstCry Parenting. Retrieved May 12, 2022, from https://parenting.firstcry.com/articles/malnutrition-and-pregnancy-risks-for-mother-and-baby/

76. *Maternal nutrition.* (2022, April 22). Maternal Nutrition. Retrieved May 12, 2022, from https://www.unicef.org/nutrition/maternal

77. *Nutrition During Pregnancy.* (n.d.). ACOG. Retrieved May 12, 2022, from https://www.acog.org/womens-health/faqs/nutrition-during-pregnancy

78. *People at Risk: Pregnant Women.* (2019, April 28). FoodSafety.Gov. Retrieved May 12, 2022, from https://www.foodsafety.gov/people-at-risk/pregnant-women\

79. *Poor nutrition during pregnancy and lactation negatively affects neurodevelopment of the offspring: evidence from a translational primate model.* (2013, August 1). PubMed Central (PMC). Retrieved May 12, 2022, from https://www.ncbi.nlm.nih.gov/pmc/articles/PMC3712549/

80.   *Pregnancy diet: What to eat and what to avoid.* (n.d.). Retrieved May 12, 2022, from https://www.medicalnewstoday.com/articles/246404

81.   *Pregnancy and prenatal vitamins.* (2020, August 19). WebMD. Retrieved May 12, 2022, from https://www.webmd.com/baby/guide/prenatal-vitamins

82. *Prenatal vitamins: Why they matter, how to choose.* (2022, April 19). Mayo Clinic. Retrieved May 12, 2022, f   r   o   m https://www.mayoclinic.org/healthy-lifestyle/pregnancy-week-by-week/in-depth/prenatal-vitamins/art-20046945

83. Schmutz, P., Hoyle, E. H., Fraser, A., & Wilson, A. N. (2019, October 10). *Food Safety for Pregnant Women & Their Babies | Home & Garden Information Center.* Home & Garden Information Center | Clemson University, South Carolina; hgic.clemson.edu. https://hgic.clemson.edu/factsheet/food-safety-for-pregnant-women-their-babies/

84.   *Undernutrition during Pregnancy.* IntechOpen (2019, January 9). Retrieved May 12, 2022, from https://www.intechopen.com/chapters/64950

85.   *Vitamins and supplements during pregnancy.* (n.d.). Pregnancy Birth and Baby. Retrieved May 12, 2022,   from

https://www.pregnancybirthbaby.org.au/vitamins-and-s
upplements-during-pregnancy

86. *What Are Prenatal Vitamins? Which to Take Before Pregnancy*. (n.d.). Planned Parenthood. Retrieved May 12, 2022, from https://www.plannedparenthood.org/learn/pregnancy/pre-pregnancy-health/what-are-prenatal-vitamins

87. Wu, G., Bazer, F. W., Cudd, T. A., Meininger, C. J., & Spencer, T. E. (2004, September 1). *Maternal Nutrition and Fetal Development | The Journal of Nutrition | Oxford Academic*. OUP Academic; academic.oup.com. https://academic.oup.com/jn/article/134/9/2169/4688801

88. *274 Tips for Baby-Proofing Your Home*. (2017, April 26). Pathways.Org. Retrieved May 13, 2022, from https://pathways.org/baby-proofing-14-tips-home/

89. *Baby Checklist: 56 Baby Essentials*. (2019, October 16). The Bump. Retrieved May 13, 2022, from https://www.thebump.com/a/checklist-baby-essentials

90. *Baby Proofing Checklist for Before Baby Can Crawl*. (2017, October 4). The bump. Retrieved May 13, 2022, from https://www.thebump.com/a/checklist-babyproofing-part-1

91. *Babyproofing Your House: A Checklist for Every Room.* (2020, September 25). Parents. Retrieved May 13, 2022, from https://www.parents.com/baby/safety/babyproofing/babyproofing-your-home-from-top-to-bottom/

92. *Birth Plans (for Parents) - Nemours KidsHealth.* (2018, June 1). Birth Plans (for Parents) - Nemours KidsHealth; kidshealth.org. https://kidshealth.org/en/parents/birth-plans.html

93. *Budgeting for New Baby: Ongoing & One-Time Expenses.* (2022, May 2). Investopedia. Retrieved May 13, 2022, from https://www.investopedia.com/articles/pf/08/budgeting-for-baby.asp

94. *Choosing a Maternity Care Provider.* (n.d.).Childbirth connection. Retrieved May 16, 2022, from http://www.childbirthconnection.org/healthy-pregnancy/choosing-a-care-provider/

95. *Choosing a healthcare provider.* (n.d.). Pregnancy Info. Retrieved May 13, 2022, from https://www.pregnancyinfo.ca/before-you-conceive/your-health-prior-to-pregnancy/choosing-a-healthcare-provider/

96. *Choosing the right health care provider for pregnancy and childbirth*. (2020, May 10). MedlinePlus Medical Encyclopedia. Retrieved May 13, 2022, from https://medlineplus.gov/ency/patientinstructions/000596.htm

97. *Employment Considerations During Pregnancy and the Postpartum Period*. (n.d) ACOG. Retrieved May 13, 2022, from https://www.acog.org/clinical/clinical-guidance/committee-opinion/articles/2018/04/employment-considerations-during-pregnancy-and-the-postpartum-period

98. *Everything You Need to Pack in Your Hospital Bag*. (2022, May 9). Babylist. Retrieved May 13, 2022, from https://www.babylist.com/hello-baby/what-to-pack-in-your-hospital-bag

99. *Health Coverage Options for Pregnant or Soon to Be Pregnant Women*. (n.d.). HealthCare.Gov. Retrieved May 13, 2022, from https://www.healthcare.gov/what-if-im-pregnant-or-plan-to-get-pregnant/

100. *Health Insurance and Pregnancy 101*. (n.d.). eHealth Insurance. Retrieved May 13, 2022, from https://www.ehealthinsurance.com/resources/guide/everything-you-need-to-know-about-health-insurance-and-pregnancy

101.   *Health and safety during pregnancy and on return to work*. (2022, April 28). Maternity Action. Retrieved May 13, 2022, from https://maternityaction.org.uk/advice/health-and-safety-during-pregnancy-and-on-return-to-work/

102.   *Hospital Bag Checklist: What to Pack in Hospital Bag*. (2019, August 12). The Bump. Retrieved May 13, 2022, from https://www.thebump.com/a/checklist-packing-a-hospital-bag

103.   *How do you prepare your older child for the separation from you while you give birth?* (n.d). Retrieved May 16, 2022, from https://www.ahaparenting.com/read/preparing-child-separation-while-birth-new-baby

104.   *How to Create Your Birth Plan: A Checklist for Parents*. (2020, July 22). Parents. Retrieved May 13, 2022, from https://www.parents.com/pregnancy/giving-birth/labor-and-delivery/checklist-how-to-write-a-birth-plan/

105.   *How to Pick a Hospital for Pregnancy & Birth*. (2020, December 9). Cleveland Clinic. Retrieved May 13, 2022, from https://health.clevelandclinic.org/how-to-choose-a-healthcare-provider-for-your-pregnancy-and-childbirth/

106.   *How to Select an OB/GYN for Your Pregnancy.*
(2022, January 6). Verywell Family. Retrieved May 13,
2022,   from
https://www.verywellfamily.com/how-to-select-an-ob-gy
n-for-your-pregnancy-5210222

107.   *Insurance When You're Pregnant.* (2020,
September 4). WebMD. Retrieved May 13, 2022, from
https://www.webmd.com/health-insurance/aca-pregnan
cy-faq

108.   *Making a birth plan - what to include, purpose,
benefits.* (n.d.). Pregnancy Birth and Baby. Retrieved May
13,   2022,   from
https://www.pregnancybirthbaby.org.au/making-a-birth
-plan

109.   *Newborn Baby Essentials: The Ultimate Baby
Checklist.* (2021, December 13). Web-Pampers-US-EN.
Retrieved   May   13,   2022,   from
https://www.pampers.com/en-us/pregnancy/preparing-f
or-your-new-baby/article/newborn-baby-checklist

110.   *New   Baby   Checklist:
Everything You Need Before Baby Arrives.* (2020,
July 1). New Parent. Retrieved May 13, 2022, from
https://newparent.com/pregnancy/new-baby-checklist/

111.   *Pack your bag for labour.* (n.d.). NHS.
Retrieved   May   13,   2022,   from

https://www.nhs.uk/pregnancy/labour-and-birth/preparing-for-the-birth/pack-your-bag-for-labour/

112.   *Preparing Your Child For A New Baby*. (n.d). Cleveland Clinic. Retrieved May 16, 2022, from https://my.clevelandclinic.org/health/articles/5185-pregnancy-preparing-children-for-the-birth-of-a-sibling

113.   *The Ultimate Baby Safety Guide*. (2017, October 26). Mom Loves Best. Retrieved May 13, 2022, from https://momlovesbest.com/health/babyproofing

114.   *Tips to choosing the right heath care provider for your pregnancy and delivery*. (2020, August 25). WebMD.   Retrieved   May   13,   2022,   from https://www.webmd.com/baby/pregnancy-choosing-obstetric-health-care-provider

115.   *What It Costs to Have and Raise a Baby*. (2020, March 19). WebMD. Retrieved May 13, 2022, f   r   o   m https://www.webmd.com/baby/what-it-costs-to-have-and-raise-a-baby

Thank you so much for reading this book. I hope you found it informative. If you did, please leave a genuine review on Amazon. This way, other pregnant mothers get to read it and benefit from it as well.